Study Skills *for* Nurses

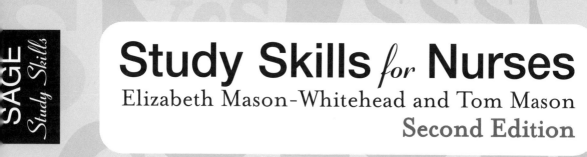

# Study Skills *for* Nurses

Elizabeth Mason-Whitehead and Tom Mason

## Second Edition

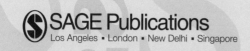

**SAGE** Publications

Los Angeles • London • New Delhi • Singapore

First edition published 2003
Reprinted 2004, 2005, 2006
This second edition published 2008

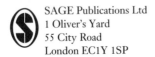

SAGE Publications Ltd
1 Oliver's Yard
55 City Road
London EC1Y 1SP

SAGE Publications Inc.
2455 Teller Road
Thousand Oaks, California 91320

SAGE Publications India Pvt Ltd
B 1/I 1 Mohan Cooperative Industrial Area
Mathura Road
New Delhi 110 044

SAGE Publications Asia-Pacific Pte Ltd
33 Pekin Street #02-01
Far East Square
Singapore 048763

**Library of Congress Control Number: 2007927713**

**British Library Cataloguing in Publication data**

A catalogue record for this book is available from the
British Library

ISBN 978-1-4129-3416-9
ISBN 978-1-4129-3417-6 (pbk)

Typeset by C&M Digitals (P) Ltd., Chennai, India
Printed in Great Britain by The Cromwell Press Ltd, Trowbridge, Wiltshire
Printed on paper from sustainable resources

Dedication
This book is dedicated to our mothers,
Rosemary Elizabeth Miller and Hilda Mason

# Contents

# List of Boxes

# List of Illustrations

# About the Authors

**Elizabeth Mason-Whitehead, PhD, BA (Hons), PGDE, RGN, RM, RHV, ONC**, is a nurse, midwife and health visitor. She has worked within these disciplines for over 30 years and her professional posts included that of midwifery sister and health visitor. After 20 years in clinical practice Elizabeth embarked upon an academic career at the University of Liverpool. Elizabeth's research, teaching and publishing interests are in the fields of social exclusion, stigma, teenage pregnancy, nurse education, research methodology and community issues. Elizabeth has published four books and over 15 journal articles. Her current post is Reader in Community Nursing and Health in the Faculty of Health and Social Care at the University of Chester.

**Tom Mason, PhD, BSc (Hons), RMN, RNMH, RGN**, is a nurse who has worked in mental health for over 30 years. He has spent approximately half this time in clinical practice and half in academic posts including research and lecturing. He has published widely on a number of related topics in mental health practice, including over 70 journal articles and 12 books. Tom is currently Professor of Mental Health and Learning Disabilities in the Faculty of Health and Social Care at the University of Chester.

# Preface

An alternative title for 'Study Skills for Nurses, Second Edition' might have been 'Mind the Gap'. Since the first edition four years ago, the gap between a number of realities and expectations continues to widen. The effect this has on the educational experience of university students and nursing students in particular is to create a sense of confusion and disappointment.

One of the most significant 'challenge gaps' that students are faced with is that their ideas and expectations of nursing, which often have their roots in childhood, are at odds with both theory and practice within their programme. For example, students just want to learn how to look after patients, get on their wards and do what they've always wanted to do – nurse! As students, your expectations are understandable and, if you have not found out already, the reality is that the process of actually becoming a nurse can appear to be unnecessarily difficult.

Another 'challenge gap' is the difference between students' and lecturers' expectations of how essays and assignments should be written and presented. In our experience, a particular issue here is referencing and this appears to cause unnecessary concern. We have attempted to address this in the second edition.

A third difference and one which brings together confusion, anger and frustration is what happens in the skills lab or classroom and how it compares to the clinical placement. This anxiety is linked to a fundamental philosophy of nursing which is now firmly rooted in evidence rather than tradition. The evidence for nursing practice is for the most part provided, disseminated and utilised by nurses themselves. The skills of studying are therefore fundamental to contemporary nursing practice. This book acknowledges that any given cohort is made up of students with a plethora of educational experiences and qualifications and who may anticipate further study with equally varying degrees of anxiety.

We also recognise that to engage fully with the profession, nurses will study for life, whether it be through educational degrees, professional qualifications or private study. Developing skills to meet new teaching methods is something which all students must strive for if they are to benefit from their programme.

We commence this second edition with a new assertion of an old argument – that if we are to be a credible profession, we must write well and publish widely. The accomplished essay that is clearly planned, appropriately referenced and professionally accurate remains a tangible benchmark of a discipline's credibility and aspirations.

As authors with a growing family and home commitments we understand the complexities of studying in environments which are less than conducive! In this book we have put forward our ideas and experiences of how you, the student, might manage these situations and how you might be supported.

In this edition we have included a new chapter for students with special needs, an acknowledgement that increasingly students who study nursing reflect the diversity of the patients and clients they care for. The concept of caring is a core principle of nursing. If students are to fulfil their potential, then the support offered to patients and clients must be extended to nurses as well.

*Elizabeth Mason-Whitehead and Tom Mason*
*University of Chester*
*April 2007*

# Acknowledgements

We would like to thank the staff and students at the University of Chester for their support during the construction of this second edition. We have been encouraged along the way by many but would particularly like to thank the Dean, Professor Mike Thomas and the Associate Dean, Dr Annette McIntosh. We would also like to thank Alison Poyner, Zoe Elliott-Fawcett and Anna Luker from Sage for their continuous encouragement throughout the process.

## 1 Introduction

**LEARNING OUTCOMES**

1. To understand the significance and implications of studying nursing within a higher education setting.
2. To be aware of the etiquette of studentship.
3. To be aware of the strengths and weaknesses of fear and confidence in study.
4. To appreciate that studying nursing is a dynamic process.
5. To know how to use this textbook to meet the needs of the individual.
6. To understand the responsibilities that students and lecturers have towards each other.

## Introduction

Throughout this book we will emphasise the practical nature of studying, which at one level may suggest that we have dismissed the importance of theory. However, this is not the case. We argue that studying comprises a set of skills that can be learnt, practised and brought together as one overall procedure, and that this approach will enhance your chances of success. In this introductory chapter we will outline the method of using this book to advance your study skills and highlight the significance of studying nursing in higher education. Being a student requires a mental attitude and a set of behaviours which are necessary if the process of studying is to be both enjoyable and successful. However, being a student often conflicts with vocational training and we will discuss some approaches to managing these difficulties. Fear and confidence will be examined in relation to these strengths and weaknesses for the student and the etiquette of being both a student and a lecturer will be outlined.

## How to Use this Book

You will get the most from this book if you work your way through it from start to finish. However, we have constructed it so that you can dip into specific chapters as you require them and to this extent they can be read independently. The book is logically constructed to reflect how you should approach the overall endeavour of studying in a modern learning environment. That is, one needs to address the practical issues of managing the home environment and the adjustments that family and friends will need to make in order to free up your time for study. The technology available to us, to assist us in studying, needs to be learnt and the voluminous amount of literature must be managed. Studying, writing, referencing and passing exams and assignments should be undertaken and the gain in knowledge needs to inform practice developments. Finally, we need to develop our ability to reflect on what we have learnt and contribute to the overall development of the profession. This cycle of learning is a continuous process and once we learn to undertake it effectively it will become a pleasurable endeavour and a rewarding experience.

We have structured the chapters so that they have a balance of text and illustrations to aid learning, and these include an opening box to include a set of 'learning outcomes' to highlight what you should have learnt by the end of the chapter. At the end of each chapter there is a box which asks you to answer some basic questions that you ought to have learnt throughout the chapter, and we provide page numbers so that you can refer to where the answer is in the chapter if needed, and a 'practical session', which sets you a few short exercises to reinforce the learning outcomes of the chapter. We have also employed two symbols throughout the chapters, one based on 'signposts' to guide you on your journey and one entitled 'learning aid' to emphasise the main points.

Chapter 2 is concerned with time management and deals with the difficult issues of learning to study in itself, and learning to study nursing as a profession. We also discuss balancing studying, working and leisure time in relation to the many and varied responsibilities that we have for other people in our lives. We have included a semester study plan that can be adapted for your own use. In Chapter 3 we outline the difficulties of managing the new information technology that is involved in modern-day studying. As information and knowledge grow, there is an ever-increasing number of sources to be searched and we now have available to us numerous software packages to help us with this. Chapter 4 specifically addresses the difficulties of managing the voluminous amount of literature that has been produced over time and the growing amount that is produced on a weekly basis. We highlight many practical suggestions as to how we can access, manage and critique this growing literature. In Chapter 5 we work through the process and structure of writing assignments, which is commonly a difficult area for students, particularly if they are new to adult study or are returning to study following a long absence. We have included a plan and checklist for writing assignments. Referencing is dealt with in Chapter 6 and this is often incorrectly considered to be either unimportant for students or a question of pedantry. We show how to reference, as well as how to manage references within the construction of written text. We have included the various referencing systems, including the APA system, which is now commonly used throughout higher education. Chapter 7 is concerned with the process of passing exams and covers this topic from the perspective of anxieties, overcoming them and sitting down to do the exam. We are mindful of the variety of theoretical assessments that students are faced with and we have therefore included OSCEs (Objective Structure Clinical Exams) and problem-based learning. In Chapter 8 we stress the importance of relating theory to practice and show how they can be viewed as separate entities or considered as one conjoint activity. Chapter 9 is a new chapter for this second edition. Its inclusion reflects the growth in students with special needs and considers how their needs can be addressed within the higher education system. Chapter 10, is concerned with the theories of reflection and its importance in modern-day nursing as a process for developing practice. We also mention how we learn from reflection and how we can improve our writing by employing it in our assignments. Finally, in Chapter 11 we deal with the issue of personal professional development and enhancing the standing of the profession of nursing itself.

# Why Study Nursing?

Nurses qualifying today do so in the knowledge that they have been successful in a course of study that has met the rigorous academic requirements of higher education. The academic ascent of nurses into colleges of higher education and universities has been a steep learning curve that previous generations of nurses would find hard to imagine. Fundamental to the growing professionalisation of nursing is a will to engage in the academic heart of evidence-based practice. For those of us who are responsible for the delivery of nurse education we must recognise the demands of higher education that nurses face, at whatever level they may be studying. These demands raise a number of issues for both students and lecturers, and we must all begin to address these issues in the quest for improved quality of nurse education.

The reasons for the increased professionalisation of nursing are reflected in the expectations of a changing society as a whole. Nurses, like many others in society, work to develop and enhance their professional knowledge base whilst simultaneously increasing their professional opportunities, status and integrity. This increase in professionalisation is also reflected in the standards laid down by the Nursing and Midwifery Council (NMC), which stipulates that all nurses must meet the CPD (continuous professional development) and PREP (post-registration education and practice) requirements. Nurses are also cognisant of the range of pressures from other groups of people. First, there are fellow professionals in medicine and the allied professions who rely on nurses to have an extended knowledge of their particular work. Second, there is also an expectation that nursing often interfaces with, and often overlaps, the work of the other professionals engaged in healthcare delivery. This belief shows the unique position of the nurse as being at the epicentre of the caring professions. Third, the growth of medical technology and medical knowledge places a profound responsibility on nurses to continually increase and build upon their own 'reservoir' of knowledge. This is essential if nurses are to continue to be critical members of the clinical team.

Fourth, successive governments since the beginning of the NHS (National Health Service) in 1948 have made an impact on some aspect of the health service, which is still considered to be one of the most highly prized structures of British life. Nurses have been forced to respond to the changing aspirations and beliefs of various governments in relation to healthcare delivery, and many of these changes have affected nurses in very significant ways. For example, consultant nurses, who have high degrees of expertise and responsibility, and are expected to be engaged in both clinical practice and research, have been introduced. Fifth, nurses do not work in a static community where illness and health remain constant. On the contrary, nurses are responding to a changing society with new social diseases such as HIV, and also a rise in some 'old' diseases as in the case of tuberculosis. For nurses to carry out their work effectively, they must have an in-depth knowledge of the causes, effects and treatment of both established and new medical conditions. Finally, and of equal importance, are the changing expectations of the population in general, and in particular when a member of the public becomes a patient. The growth of lay health knowledge amongst the general public, from the literature, the media and the Internet, has given rise to a more informed, discerning and critical society. The implications for nurses are clear and include the need to deliver a high standard of care that is both evidence-based and patient-focused.

Nursing is one of the more recent disciplines to enter higher education, but the rules and regulations, standards and quality, and principles and values of academic life are the same for all courses and for all students. No matter what subject is taught in higher education, the quality of the teaching, as well as the quality of the learning, should be the same. Put another way, a first-class honours in one subject should equate with a first-class honours in another. Thus, the quality of the student is paramount. As some students who wish to study nursing, either those new to nursing or nurses returning to study, may not have had the opportunities to learn how to study in modern higher educational settings, this book will help to address this.

The development of the nursing educational ethos has also included a shift in understanding the relationship between nursing and 'science'. The notion of 'science' involves ideas about logical assumptions, cause and effect, and the production of evidence. In modern-day nursing we are increasingly under pressure to base our practice on evidence rather than tradition, and to be able to explicate rational nursing action rather than engage in ritualistic behaviour. The term evidence-based practice may well be viewed, and abused, as a convenient buzzword by some, but its import cannot be stressed enough in contemporary healthcare settings. It is important for a number of reasons: first, that the delivery of modern healthcare is a rational process, which balances patient needs with available resources, and there is no room for wasteful practices, including nursing care. Second, as professionals, nurses are accountable for their actions and the public expects them to be highly trained and highly skilled. Furthermore, it is expected that nurses maintain their professional knowledge and expertise through updating and lifelong learning. Third, nursing knowledge needs to be grounded in evidence as our contemporary society is becoming increasingly litigious, and nurses are being made more responsible for the delivery of care. We hope that this book makes the study of nursing a more pleasant endeavour and a more effective enterprise.

# Different Students, Different Needs

We begin with the assumption that whatever your reasons for wishing to study nursing, every student of learning who reads any part of this book will be working towards the same objective: a successful outcome. In our experience, we know that the journey to such success can either be chaotic, tortuous and more a question of luck than judgement, or it can be planned, anticipated and enjoyable. This text is about how to achieve the latter. We aim to embrace all students who are studying nursing and we are appreciative of the wide diversity of people embarking on nursing studies, either as new students of nursing, those qualified nurses who are returning to practice after a break in service or those qualified nurses who are now undertaking further qualifications.

This text will be used differently by students, depending upon the experience they have and the course they are attending. For example, it may be that the 'aids to learning' will be more beneficial to those students with the least experience of modern-day study. We envisage that for the most experienced students this book will provide an up-to-date and accessible reference source for study skills and provide practical ideas and innovations to overcome the many problems of studying in contemporary times.

The different levels of expertise, and the experience that students bring, is matched by the many contrasting lifestyles that they have. Indeed, a typical cohort of diploma/degree students is made up of school leavers, graduates, people who have already qualified in one particular occupation such as teaching, those who have been prevented from nurse training because of family commitments, and those students who have worked as nursing assistants and now wish to pursue a nursing qualification. This usually makes the student group rich and lively. There are other differences, for example, gender (unfortunately nursing is still a female dominated profession with fewer than five male students in most cohorts of 100) and culture (regrettably nursing is still underrepresented in ethnic minorities). As authors we recognise the demanding lifestyles led by many people who study nursing. As nursing is predominantly a female profession these may include the responsibilities that many women have as the principal carer within their household, and, where possible, throughout this book we offer practical help for those with wide commitments.

We recognise that not only does each identified group of people present particular study challenges, but within groups every individual person comes forward with their own needs, strengths and limitations. Furthermore, it is important that students take time to understand themselves and to recognise the particular help that they may need. There is no shame in not knowing something but there is shame in not wanting to learn. For example, in our experience the lack of confidence amongst nurses who are returning to practice is a common theme that runs through most courses, and this is often a major hurdle that must be overcome in order for them to succeed with their assignments, preparing for exams and general course of study.

We are also aware, as are the majority of universities and colleges, that there are a few students who experience specific difficulties in learning. For example, there are people who have dyslexia and require additional or special help from personal and academic tutors. In addition to this we encourage those students to seek advice from the student support service of their own institution. Students often think that because they have a learning need they should keep quiet about it – nothing could be further from the truth! We remind all students studying nursing that those involved in teaching and delivering nursing courses are committed to working with students to ensure that they achieve their full potential (see Chapter 9).

## Learning Aid

Identify your learning needs and make a plan to address them as soon as you can. You will gain most from your course if you satisfy your own requirements.

We emphasise that those students who are experiencing any difficulties should see their tutors as soon as possible. Ignoring the problem will not make it go away (see Chapter 9).

As nursing lecturers ourselves we have heard many stories (and indeed we have some of our own stories!) of how some students have achieved their goals, with assignments being handed in with a minute to spare, and some students claiming to have handed assignments in when they haven't! In this text we work with students to give them a smooth and successful passage, at whatever level of study they are at, with the aim of trying to make studying a more enjoyable enterprise. However, we have to address the main fear that all students face, which is failing an assignment or exam. Of course this does happen, and students too usually have a story to tell regarding this, but in this text we will offer numerous strategies that, if undertaken, will make failing less likely.

## Early Problems?

Be proactive about any difficulties.
Do not ignore the problem.
Get help.

# Nursing Students are Integral to the University Population

Today's nursing student is one student amongst many other student groups in higher education. Nursing courses in these settings must satisfy the requirements of both the Nursing Midwifery Council and the relevant institute of higher education or university, which have their own set of standards. Not only are student nurses required to meet the national standards, but they are comparable with colleagues in the other disciplines of, say, English, Mathematics, Biology, and so on, and must meet these standards also. Furthermore, the academic standard of a single university or college should be comparable to that of all other academic institutes and reach the required level that is acceptable nationally. What does this mean for students of nursing studies? In Chapter 7 we discuss the criteria that are required for each level of achievement, and we outline what is required from students in order to achieve this. One of the tasks assigned to lecturers in any field of study is to convey to the student the ethos of studying their topic in a higher educational setting, and many students of nursing are surprised at the change in dynamic and the expectations that are placed upon them. The most obvious example of the academic work required from today's students lies in the submission of assignments, which now must be research-led and supported by relevant literature. This is often new to nursing students. Therefore, the use of evidence, and the ability to employ references is a fundamental study skill, which is now crucial for all students in higher education, including students of nursing studies.

The changing dynamic of nurse education often surprises many student nurses, not only those returning to practice, who may not be used to research-led practice, but often new students, who may have the belief that nursing is about being at the patient's bedside and assume that there is little more to it than that. The task of nurse educators is to endorse the view that nursing is about wishing to care for people who are sick but it is also about being a highly skilled and accountable professional. To become such a professional requires rigorous assessments and an ability to communicate to other professionals in an articulate and competent manner. Today, professionalism is at the heart of good nursing, where research-led practice and clear verbal and written communication skills are essential. The changing dynamic of nurse education involves a balance between nursing professionalism and academic rigour. This is not an easy task but must be achieved if nurses are to be successful in higher educational settings.

## Feel that Nursing is Changing?

Increased professionalisation.
Higher expectations of society.
Increased accountability.

Students new to nursing studies are becoming increasingly involved in different innovations of learning and assessment of students' work. As nurse educators we continually strive to develop teaching and assessing methods that can be built upon the more formal and traditional styles that students are used to. It is important that we deliver a programme that allows students not only to learn 'facts' but to express themselves and learn in a creative and proactive manner. Students will usually come across three styles of teaching and assessing, which they may not be familiar with. First is group work as a style of teaching. Students may be taught in teaching slots of one, two or three hours. A three-hour slot of formal teaching can be arduous for all concerned and is likely to be broken up into smaller sections. Group work usually follows a standard lecture, and for the final hour of the session the class may be asked to break into groups to discuss a particular subject arising from the lecture. For example, the lecture may be on discrimination and stigmatisation and the group work may be looking at the ways in which nurses can work towards reducing discrimination in the healthcare profession. Students need to develop good communication skills in working together to produce a short presentation at the end of the session to their colleagues. New students frequently find these tasks daunting, but in our experience confidence grows very quickly with practice. Second, students may be required to give a presentation as part of a seminar. This may be an individual effort or as part of a group, and the seminar may be part of the module assessment. Speaking in front of people can be a very daunting task for many people, particularly when they are unused to the experience. As mentioned above, the more it is undertaken the easier it becomes, and confidence will increase. Third, 'problem-based learning' (PBL) has found its way into the nursing curriculum because it is a tool that helps nurses prepare for their clinical practice. PBL has been explained as:

An instructional method in which students work in small groups to gain knowledge and acquire problem-solving skills. A major characteristic of PBL is that the problem is presented to the student *before* the material has been learned rather than after, as in the more traditional 'problem-solving approach'. A second notable feature is the context in which students are likely to encounter the given (or similar) problem in real life. (Wilkie, 2000: 11)

Students may feel a little anxious about, and even hostile towards, 'new' teaching methods and different methods of assessment and we suggest that they take time to discuss their concerns with fellow students and staff. Usually, different methods of teaching come as a welcome change because they allow students to learn in a more creative way. Finally, there are practical exams known as OSCEs (Objective Structural Clinical Exams) and these are becoming increasingly popular in testing students' ability to perform clinical procedures such as reading a blood pressure and taking a blood sample. All of these methods of assessment support, and in some instances replace, conventional means of assessment. However, it is the assignment and the examination that continue to be the foundation of theoretical assessments for nursing programmes. (Problem-based learning and other theoretical assessments are discussed in Chapter 5.)

## Being a Student

The common perception of the lifestyle of a student varies considerably. This can range from a student who is perceived to be constantly partying to the studious bookworm burning the midnight oil. Despite this difference of opinion there is one thing that is generally agreed upon and that is at whatever age we start our student days the experience offers a specialness that cannot be captured at any other time of our lives. This belief is rooted in the expectations of student life, where entering a new culture offers the prospect of meeting new friends, facing new challenges, and experiencing new learning opportunities, which will result in a rewarding qualification and a satisfying career. Again, there is a balance to be drawn between study, rest and play, with each one offering the potential for academic growth and development. You should not leave your student days feeling unfulfilled. Maximise your potential in all areas of life.

## Want a Student's Life?

Balance between work, rest and play.
You will get out of it what you put in.

Students who embark upon a vocational course, such as medicine, physiotherapy or nursing studies, have a unique experience of carrying the burden of having two 'masters', the college or university of study and the governing body of their chosen profession (see Illustration 1:1).

The additional rules and regulations implemented by professional bodies often cause students to feel stifled, and restrict them from the academic freedom that their non-vocational fellow students appear to have. Nursing students quickly realise that the pressures of the programme to fulfil the stipulated number of hours mean that

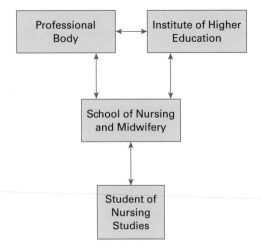

**Illustration 1:1    The College Framework in Relation to the Nursing Student**

theoretical days in college are packed with lectures, with little time for additional scholarly endeavour or college activities. This disadvantage is further exacerbated by students being away from college for clinical placements, and who may then find it difficult to join college sports teams and social events. Nurses studying in higher education may feel excluded from the main student body. For example, nursing students do not always follow the college academic year and they can be in class when other students are away. To their dismay they frequently find campus banks, libraries, bookshops and cafés closed, and understandably feel undervalued by this. Some nursing courses extend into the evening when the campus is empty, dark and uninviting. Incorrectly, other student groups may feel that nursing is merely a practical enterprise and does not carry academic weight. These issues must be faced if nurses are to feel integrated and valued in college life, and part of this involves engaging with being a student in a mature fashion.

## Learning Aid

What do you understand by the term student? What do you expect to get out of being a student?

What will you put into it?

The above paragraphs paint a rather arduous picture for nursing students, but there are ways of overcoming these challenges and the sections throughout the book deal with this. Ultimately, we accept that studying nursing does have difficulties in a higher educational setting, but once these are addressed the rewards of studying nursing are rich, both intellectually and clinically.

## A Student of Nursing in Higher Education?

Having to satisfy two masters.
Working around lifestyles.
Intellectually and clinically demanding.

Finally, being a student means, of course, that you have to study. At the outset of your course your knowledge of your subject will be scant, with perhaps only limited knowledge of nursing gained from anecdotes, television, and so on. We would suggest that you consider your mind to be like an empty 'reservoir' at the start of your course and that this 'reservoir' requires to be filled with knowledge. Throughout your course you will learn from being taught in the classroom or lecture theatre and in the clinical areas. However, you will also learn by reading in your own time and it is this reading that contributes significantly to filling the 'reservoir'. Take every spare moment that you can and read. Read books, journals, reports, articles – in fact anything and everything that you can, which is related to nursing. The more you fill your 'reservoir' of knowledge, the more you will have to draw upon when the time comes for your exams or assignments. You are responsible for filling your 'reservoir' of knowledge. No one else is.

## Expectations of Students and Lecturers

Students have a wide range of people that they can draw upon from within their college. However, before we discuss the individual relationships you can have with 'significant people' in detail, we have provided an illustration of how the nursing student is part of the school and the college in Illustration 1:1 on page 10.

Unless nursing students have previously undergone a period of study in an institute of higher education, it is likely that their previous formal experience of the student–teacher relationship will have been at secondary school. In these cases student nurses may commence their college programme with the expectations that the relationship that they will have with the lecturer will be similar to that of the teacher–pupil relationship that they remember from school. The reality is, of course, very different and the transition from learning in a school to being an adult student in higher education can be a shock for the new student! The result is that lecturers and students can be both surprised and disappointed with each other's behaviour, with each complaining that the other just doesn't know how to be a proper 'student' or 'lecturer'. We believe that this unhappy situation arises because the formal rules and regulations for students, which are explicit in contracts, programmes and module handbooks, do not inform the student of the *unwritten* rules of studentship. These are the informal rules, which students must learn for themselves through error and experience. They are often implicit but can be summarised under the heading of student etiquette, and both knowing and implementing these will give the student a smoother passage through college. Some of these rules can be seen in Box 1:1.

## Box 1:1   The Expectations and Etiquette of Students' Relationship with their Tutors

- Treat your tutor with respect and courtesy at all times; your tutor should do the same to you.
- Make an appointment to see your new personal/academic tutor as soon as possible.
- Don't expect to see your tutor without an appointment, unless you have a problem that requires urgent attention.
- Don't thrust work into your tutor's hand and expect them to mark it immediately.
- Always knock on the tutor's door before entering their office.
- Anticipate and make appointments well in advance of submission deadlines.
- You are expected to see your personal/academic tutor for tutorials; however, it is acceptable to approach another tutor if your tutor is not available.
- Don't expect your tutor to give last-minute appointments to check work that has to be submitted the following day.
- Inform your tutor in advance if possible, if you have to rearrange a scheduled appointment.
- Plan your work before your tutorial, have the criteria of what you want from the tutorial beforehand and stick to the agenda.
- Where possible, submit work to your tutor before your planned meeting. Ensure that you have a copy of the work that you have submitted and also ensure that your work is clear and legible.
- Take notes during the meeting.
- Make an appointment to see your tutor for a follow-up tutorial if required.

The unwritten rules of being a student also extend to how one should behave both in class and within the college as a whole. Whilst some students may be surprised that this information needs to be expressed, other students would not be. We do not prescribe a particular code of behaviour, but rather ask students to reflect on their own actions and ask what they consider to be appropriate behaviour. For example, do students feel it is acceptable for lecturers to chew gum during the lecture? If not, is it acceptable for the students in class to chew? We anticipate that some students will feel that this behaviour is unacceptable from both the lecturer and the student, and others may not. However, it is this type of behaviour that suggests the areas of the unspoken code regarding the etiquette of study in higher education. They are often a question of manners and employing a respect for others.

- Have consideration for your colleagues and lecturer in the classroom situation; consider and reflect if your behaviour is appropriate – for example, eating, drinking, chewing gum, walking out during the middle of a lecture, arriving late and talking during the session.
- As an adult learner, your experience should be both proactive and interactive, and you are therefore expected to read around your subject before and after the lecture.
- It is not acceptable to hawk your work around the school asking every lecturer if they will check your assignment and tell you if it will pass!

Etiquette is a two-way process. We are mindful that this process involves professional standards of the academic institute and the obligations of the student. It is obligatory for the college to provide the highest level of instruction and for the student to engage in their studies. Problems occur when the expectations that each has of the other person's role in the study process are unfulfilled. Knowing one's own role is important, but knowing what can be expected of others is paramount to good study practice.

The following points illustrate the major expectations that students can have of the lecturing staff:

- To be treated with respect and courtesy at all times.
- To have access to academic staff and to be able to make appointments with their personal/academic tutor.
- To have access to the college student support department.
- To have support from the clinical setting from named mentors.
- To have access to information on programmes, courses, modules, assessments and examinations.
- To have the module content completed within the designated time.
- To have empathic personal tutors who will deal with personal issues sensitively.

- To have any issues of grievance taken seriously.
- To have from the lecturer a summary of the tutorial at the end of the session, covering the issues discussed, including any difficulties, progress made, planned work, and, where appropriate, the next tutorial appointment.

## Being a Student?

Understand your role as a student.
Understand the roles of others in the enterprise.
Understand that etiquette is a two-way process.
Adhere to formal and informal rules of behaviour.

# Fear and Confidence

Both fear and confidence are natural states, which prepare us to respond to a particular situation or event that we face. Without them we would be less prepared and therefore, in evolutionary terms, less likely to survive. They have both physical as well as psychological elements to them, which work together to create the characteristic emotions that accompany them. We should accept both fear and confidence as part and parcel of life and consider that a little bit of both is probably a good thing. Problems are encountered, however, when they become extreme and they then negatively impact on our ability to perform as well as we might like.

What is fearful to one person is not necessarily fearful to another and the situations that create anxiety are usually dependent upon the amount of experience that we have had in dealing with these situations. In terms of studying, it may be that you are new to this in adult life or returning to it after a long period of time, and this is causing you some anxiety. It may be that it is managing your time, navigating the library or dealing with the computers that are creating some degree of fear. In any event, it is usually the sitting of exams that creates the most fear, in most of us. Whatever it is that is causing the most anxiety, the first step to overcoming it is to accept that it is real and important to you. Similarly, the anxiety felt by others is also real and important to them. The worst comment to be heard when someone is expressing their anxiety is 'oh, you'll be all right'. This comment rarely helps to relieve any real anxiety and is more likely to give the impression that the extent of concern has not been grasped. There are some things that you can do to help you overcome your fear and the main one revolves around familiarity. The more you become familiar with something the less fearful you become of it. So, if the library, for example, causes you the greater concern, then spending more and more time in there, looking for books and searching for journals, will tend to ease the anxiety. At the outset of your course build up a network of 'friends' that you can work with, travel with, have a coffee with, go to the library with, etc., whilst you are at college, and when anxieties build up talk to others about this. Also, learn to listen to others' worries as well. You will probably have been allocated a personal tutor and/or an academic tutor when you started college so you can make an appointment with either of these and talk to them about your anxieties. If it is sitting exams that causes you angst, then we deal with this in Chapter 7. Fear and anxiety are, as we have said, a reaction to something, so the 'something' needs to be addressed. Therefore, tackle the problem head-on, as early as possible, by undertaking a plan of attack on whatever is causing the fear. Box 1:2 outlines the framework for the plan of attack and should be worked through for each area of anxiety that is identified.

Confidence, on the other hand, does not produce all the above negative feelings associated with fear but can be just as incapacitating unless it is controlled. If you approach your study correctly you should come to a stage where you feel confident that you can produce what is required and to a good standard. However, overconfidence can lead to misunderstanding what is needed, not appreciating the difficulties, and underestimating the problem. Overconfidence can lead to arrogance, which in turn narrows the mind and causes a lack of focus. Therefore, getting the balance right is crucial to being an effective student.

## Box 1:2    Plan of Attack for Problem Solving

### What is the Problem?

- Write down what you think the problem or situation is that is causing you to feel anxious (for example, library, computers, assignments).
- Now write down what specific aspects of the problem or situation are causing you the greatest concern (for example, searching books, word-processing, grammar).

### What Would be Your Best and Worst Outcome?

- Write down what you would like as your best outcome (for example, to access the books, produce a neatly presented project, write a good assignment).
- Write down what your worst-case scenario would be (for example, to be unable to find the required books, be unable to use the software, produce bad assignments, look bad in front of others).

*(Continued)*

*(Continued)*

### What Resources do I Need to Address the Problem?

- Write down what resources you need to address the problem (for example, a librarian to teach me, someone with knowledge to teach me word-processing, a book that gives me information on writing).

### What are the Priorities in Addressing the Problem?

- Write down what needs to be done immediately (for example, speak to the librarian).
- Write down what needs to be done later (for example, contact the IT department).

### What are my Options?

- Write down a number of options available to you in addressing the problem (for example, to go to the library, practise accessing books, ask a librarian to teach you, ask a knowledgeable friend).

### What are my Feelings about Addressing the Problem?

- Write down how you feel about addressing the problem, at this moment in time (for example, anxious but keen to get it sorted).
- Write down how you think you will feel once the problem is addressed (for example, will feel good and pleased).

### What am I Going to Do About It Now?

- Write down a priority list of things that you need to do to address the problem (for example, to phone librarian, allocate some time in your diary, go to the library, speak to a friend).
- Tick them off as you do them.

## Fearful or Confident?

Both are natural states.
Understand them to control them.
Address fear.
Do not get overconfident.

# Conclusions

We conclude this first chapter by reminding our readers to bear in mind three significant issues that are crucial to achieving success in the study of nursing. First, we ask students, irrespective of their level of academic attainment, to take time to consider their own lifestyles and to plan carefully their study time whilst fulfilling their commitments to others. Second, we ask students to think about what kind of student they aspire to be and to work towards their objectives, using all the support and help that is offered from the college and their school. Finally, we appreciate that acquiring study skills takes time, but once the above systems and ideas are understood then the experience of studying nursing will be enjoyable and successful.

## SUMMARY POINTS OF CHAPTER 1

- Use the book as an aid to learning.
- The study of nursing in higher education is important for both pesonal and professional reasons.
- Being a student entails a good attitude towards studying and a set of behaviours to accompany it.
- Fear and confidence are natural responses and should be managed appropriately.
- There is an etiquette involved in the learning experience, which includes both student and tutor.

# Test Your Study Skills ...

1. What are the main problems for vocational students in higher education? (see pages 9–11)

2. When does fear or anxiety begin to affect your study? (see pages 14–15)

3. What are the main problems with overconfidence? (see page 15)

4. What do you understand by student etiquette? (see pages 11–14)

5. What do the learning symbols mean to you? (see pages 5–12)

## Practical Session ...

At the outset of your study make sure that you:

1. Organise your stationery for study.

2. Acquire the module handbooks.

3. Obtain a copy of the college rules and regulations.

4. Make yourself aware of the college layout and facilities.

5. Attend the library skills sessions.

# 2 How to Manage Time Effectively

## LEARNING OUTCOMES

1. To understand the time management challenges that apply to all students when embarking upon a programme of study.
2. To understand the time management challenges that apply to students of nursing studies.
3. To understand the importance of balancing study time with other commitments.
4. To be able to develop a personal study plan.

## Introduction

Time is a finite commodity, with 24 hours in a day and seven days in a week, and it is merely what we choose to do in that time that governs our time management. However, we all have various things that we have to do and these are often priorities that are difficult to adjust. This chapter is concerned with suggestions regarding how we can balance our professional and personal activities in life and how to find time for effective studying. We will argue that there are skills involved in managing time and these include managing busy households, prioritising commitments and fulfilling responsibilities towards others. Studying is often a lone endeavour, but it also often needs the help of others by adjusting some aspect of their lives.

## Finding Time to Study

We begin this chapter with the acknowledgement that all of us have experience of managing our own time but that this may be undertaken informally and with little forward planning or strategic thought. Through our experience of managing our own study time we have built up a repertoire of ideas and practical study skills for both new nursing students and those returning to study. Studying is very much a personal endeavour and there are as many different styles of study as there are people who are engaged in the process. We have all probably met someone who appears to be well organised in all aspects of their lives, who has a clear desk with everything neatly tidied, filed and folded, and who appears to circumscribe work time, leisure time, family time and study time in a harmonious balance. We can contrast this person with another student who appears chaotic and totally disorganised. They are frequently late, always running, chasing and looking for something that they cannot find. They lose handouts, misplace projects and usually have a bag of jumbled books and articles, which appear as a mass of muddled papers. Their desks are mountainous areas of cluttered documents with little writing space. Which one of these two extremes do you more closely resemble? Where on the continuum do you most closely fit?

We cannot prescribe a particular style for you as it is clearly a personal matter and should fit with what you feel is best for you. However, what we can say is that whatever style you choose, it should be one that is based on organisation, clear thinking and sound planning. Time is valuable to all of us and we do not want to waste it by disorganised working or studying. We suggest that you understand yourself and your lifestyle before planning your study, so take a little time and consider the style of studying that suits you best and the extent of motivation that you have. Be realistic about this and assess your experience of studying. Remember that time is finite, and an honest reflection of your priorities, needs and ability to satisfy these is the best policy.

In the previous chapter we acknowledged the wide diversity of students who are at any one time studying nursing, at whatever level that may be, and the many individual styles that they bring. By the same token, we appreciate the varying experiences that people have of managing time, and that some will be better than others at this task. The differences in such experiences are vast, from the recent school leaver becoming a student at university who is used to balancing study time and a social life, to a parent becoming a student who is used to balancing the obligations of home, family, job and social pursuits. Mature students are frequently astounded when their younger and 'freer' colleagues assert that they do not have time for study! It is our experience that whatever the commitments, students will always protest, saying that there is never enough time, and indeed there never is!

Throughout our lives we use time differently, and this usually differs according to our age. Each period of our lives entails different commitments and it is these commitments that require careful consideration when we are embarking upon a life-changing event, such as attending a course of study. It is unlikely to be the case that you can incorporate a new course of study into an already busy life without changing the re-prioritisation of other commitments.

## Learning Aid

Attempting to study as well as fulfilling all other commitments in your life will probably lead to a reduction in the quality of everything. Make a list of all your commitments and include your course of study, work, family and leisure. Identify which are priorities and which can be shelved for the period of your study.

All individuals should be respected and we recognise that their commitments are both unique and important to them. What is a priority to one person may not be a priority to another.

We begin with the general issues of studying in relation to time management that are pertinent to all students. A question frequently asked by students is how much time will I need for studying? This is an impossible question to give an exact answer to as it very much depends on the individuals involved. As we have stated above, everyone has different needs, irrespective of their programme of study. All students should take time to make a thorough and comprehensive plan of their course of study, ensuring that they incorporate reading, making notes, writing assignments, revision and sitting exams. This plan should be pinned up on a wall so that you can refer to it without looking for it and you can see the progress through the course. We recommend that students should take some time to read every day and that they ensure that their study skills continue to be practised throughout their course. For some students this may mean developing their computer skills and for others it may entail revising their referencing technique. Students are advised to anticipate and plan their assignments and examination work well in advance, and to identify the sub-components of these and make individual plans for each. For most people, creating large blocks of time immediately before examinations or assignment submission dates is difficult and can lead to disaster!

## Learning Aid

Identifying a block of time shortly before the deadline is a risky practice, as something usually happens to absorb it, leaving you in desperate straits. Make a realistic plan.
The plan should cover your entire course.
Pin it up so all family members/partners/flatmates can see it.

It is with this in mind that we strongly advocate that students plan well in advance and allocate time throughout the entire course of their study. This can be achieved by diarising key dates in the programme such as when assignments need to be submitted and examinations sat. We also suggest that you make appointments to see your personal/academic tutors early in your course and plan time for tutorials, where work can be commented upon with enough time for feedback.

## The Specific Issues of Studying Nursing

The 'special-ness' of studying nursing is a theme that we will maintain throughout this book. In the previous chapter we discussed the difficulties of studying a vocational course in a higher educational setting, which revolves around the fact that students have two masters, that of their professional body as well as their institute of study. In this section we claim that the time management aspect of studying nursing also has unique characteristics that students must address if they are to achieve a successful outcome.

The specific issues relating to studying nursing appear to fall into two main areas. First, the shift system presents particular challenges for students. Students are expected to study, whether it be for exams, assignments or work related to their particular clinical area, whilst on their placement. Managing time around the shift system is a new experience for many students, particularly in relation to organising other commitments, for example, studying at different times of the day to fit in with shift patterns, which we discuss in greater depth in the next section. In addition to this, students find studying whilst on clinical placements both physically and emotionally very tiring. The stamina required for undertaking these activities necessitates that a student maintains both physical and intellectual health. At this point we do not intend to outline a health programme but merely suggest that students reflect on their lifestyle in relation to their demanding roles.

## Learning Aid

Students find studying whilst on clinical placement very tiring and do not always achieve their planned goals.

Second, many students are confronted with having to study subjects which they may find emotionally difficult. These occasions usually occur when students have a partner, relative or friend who has suffered the particular condition that is being studied. Students often feel confused by, on the one hand, wishing to understand the subject and, on the other, having sad thoughts regarding the suffering that their loved one experienced (or is experiencing). It is at these times that we suggest that students take guidance from both their lecturers and from their personal/academic tutors.

## Find Studying Tough?

Physically demanding.
Keep healthy.
Nursing can be emotionally draining.
Ensure you have a support network.

# How to Balance the Responsibilities of a Busy Life and Study Effectively

This section discusses how we can aim to balance our commitments and fulfil our course requirements by addressing the needs of both others and ourselves. We do not pretend that it is anything other than one of the most complex and difficult aspects of studying, as some students do not receive the full support of others. Indeed, one of the reasons why students do not complete, or are not successful in their studies is because they are overwhelmed by what is asked of them from home, work and college. Consequently, it is the study that frequently suffers. Clearly, we cannot provide individual answers for particular students' circumstances, but through our own experiences, and those of students and fellow lecturers, we can offer guidelines and suggestions that students may be able to adapt to their own particular circumstances.

## Learning Aid

Managing study time effectively is one of the most complex of all study skills. Those students who are so overwhelmed by their many responsibilities may not complete their course or fail their theoretical work.

The fundamental rules of balancing commitments and responsibilities are to anticipate problems, communicate with others, plan thoroughly, implement proactively, evaluate effectively and amend accordingly. Make a list of the main problems that you think will arise in the course of your study and prioritise them with the most serious at the top. Then go through each problem and identify who are the people that you need to communicate with in order either to acquire information or to discuss the problem. It is often the case that once we have discussed the problem with others we can negotiate a solution. This may not be a perfect one but at least it may ease the situation. You can use the six-fold plan as outlined in Illustration 2:1 for each problem that you anticipate.

The more commitments that students have, the earlier this six-fold plan should begin. Indeed, many of these responsibilities can be organised before the course of study begins. For example, childcare can take some time to arrange and a number of significant issues have to be accounted for to ensure that everyone involved is comfortable with the situation. We consider the issues involved with arranging childcare later in the chapter.

| Aspects of Plan | Rationale |
| --- | --- |
| Anticipate | Think ahead and identify what problems you think that you might encounter. Make a priority list. |
| Communicate | Identify who you need to talk to in order to address the problem. This might be the person who is causing you the problem or others who may be able to offer help/advice. |
| Plan | Make a plan of action to address the problem. This might include who and when you are going to talk with and the best time to do so. |
| Implement | Put the plan into action. Do not put it off. |
| Evaluate | What was the result of the implementation? Was the problem solved or did it make things worse? |
| Amend | Change the plan and have another attempt. Try something different. |

**Illustration 2:1   Six-Fold Plan For Problem Solving**

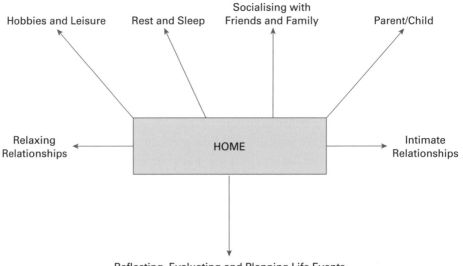

**Illustration 2:2   Activities within the home**

## A Juggling Act?

List all your commitments and prioritise.
Plan extensively.
Organise early.

We now move on to examine how each 'domain' of our responsibilities carries particular characteristics. Within the following sections, we examine the nature of these challenges and how they can be overcome.

## Box 2:1   Topics for Family/Partner Meetings

- Make time to communicate with members of your household.
- Inform your family/partner about the course dates, time and outcome.
- Have as much information about the course as possible, which will allow you to
  plan ahead.
- Discuss your plans in relation to those of others and be respectful of the com-
  mitments of others.
- Consider the significant planned events of the home, such as a wedding or chris-
  tening, and work towards attending these functions.
- Discuss the ways in which small and large changes will need to be made within
  the home to fulfil the requirements of the course.
- Discuss where within the home you might study.
- Discuss the times you might study.
- Students and their family/partners will find a timetable illustrating everyone's
  commitments useful.

## Home Life

We begin with the assumption that for the majority of students 'home' is their base. Of
course, students who are studying away from their family may have a temporary home
near their college and probably aim to visit their families at weekends and holidays.
Illustration 2:2 serves to remind us of the extent to which home life has an impact upon

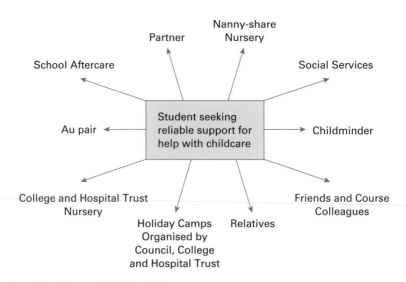

**Illustration 2:3   Support with childcare**

our decision making. For most of us, whatever form it takes, home life is a significant part of our own personal world.

Today, we often hear, and also experience, how members of households do not always meet together as often as they would wish. The reasons for this are complex but they include children growing up and leading more independent lives, longer working days and people in and out of the house at different times. Consequently, regular meetings at breakfast, lunch or supper are not always possible and messages that get passed around the family may be misinterpreted or forgotten. To address this, we advocate that students bring together the people who are significant to them in their lives and have regular, but not too frequent, meetings. These people may be their immediate family, partners or flatmates. How often students have such meetings will depend upon their particular circumstances, but Box 2:1 gives guidance to the content of these meetings.

A major issue in undertaking a course of study is the redistribution of household chores. Frequently, the student of nursing studies is also the main carer and housekeeper in the home. As lecturers we have heard many stories of partners not being able, or willing, to adjust their home life and having 'traditional' expectations of their roles. The demands of a nursing course can threaten these established practices, and may cause tensions in the home. First, the anticipated requirements of the family and partner may be undermined, where the student can no longer carry out the household duties as they did before they began their studies. We appreciate that many family members may not be accustomed to having to do those chores previously done by others. New situations take some time to get used to. Indeed, students who are also married, and may have children, are often worried that they will not be at home as frequently as they were to undertake their usual household tasks. So, if this is a problem, then communicate this to the family members, make a plan to take account of the tasks, implement it and evaluate it accordingly. Second, a nursing course with an intake of students will bring an introduction into new cultures and new social networks. Meeting people of different ages, and from a variety of backgrounds, will offer diverse experiences, which can prompt students to reconsider their attitudes and values, and that which was agreeable before may no longer be acceptable now. This may lead to family and friends stating that 'you have changed since starting that course'. Be prepared for this.

## Home Life Commitments?

Home life is important.
Others are important.
You are important.
A balance is important.
Communication is important.

We are mindful that the separation of parents from their children, for however short a period, is often emotionally difficult, particularly when the children are young. Students (and lecturers!) frequently express their guilt and feelings of missing their children and for some this will be the first occasion that children have been separated from their parents. If you are one of these parents, we can assure you that your first day on your nursing programme will be full of emotion and you will not be the only one calling your childminder at every opportunity!

We can also assure you that as the pattern of study and childminding becomes established, the easier the process will become. We also appreciate that there may be some teething problems, whether it be a telephone call to say a favourite toy has been forgotten or difficulty adjusting to a new environment. We do strongly suggest that students have a practice day(s), so that everyone involved can become used to the situation before the course begins. Illustration 2:3 will help students clarify their thoughts in deciding whom they can approach and where they can go for help with childminding.

It is important to reward children, and partners, for their role in adjusting to your course. So, have a series of treats and plan to spend some time with them. Box 2:2 is an *aide-mémoire* to help students anticipate and plan the needs of children whilst they are studying.

## Box 2:2 *Aide-mémoire* to Assist in Choosing Childcare

- If students do not know prospective carers, we advise that they take up their references.
- A list of registered childminders can be obtained from the local social services.
- We suggest that students seeking childminding should contact their local social services, who can provide a list of registered childminders; read local papers; visit libraries and visit the student union in their college and the hospital trust.
- We suggest that students hold a family meeting to discuss the childcare options.
- Students should read carefully the information provided on crèches, nurseries and childminders and ensure that all their questions are answered to their satisfaction.
- A trial run will help establish transport times, requirements for the day and give time for everyone to become accustomed to the new situation.
- Ensure that all documentation is available: for example, immunisation certificates and contactable telephone numbers.
- We suggest that students approach at least one family friend or relative who can be contacted by the carer if the student or partner is unavailable.

## Learning Aid

Do you feel comfortable with your childminding arrangements? Have you followed up all references and checks?

Anxieties over children are common.

Plan early.

Talk to the children.

Organise a support network.

Have a contingency plan.

## Caring for other vulnerable groups

In the previous section we discussed the considerations to be taken into account when caring for children whilst studying. We are also aware that many students care for other vulnerable people and that they may be a more diverse group of people of various ages and with differing needs. They may be partners, family members or close friends. They may be older and frail parents or children with special needs, or they may be sick or injured family members. Each person who is being cared for by a student will have very individual needs. Box 2:3 offers some practical tips for students who have to organise care for their relatives/friends.

## Box 2:3   Practical Help for Carers of People with Special Needs

- If it is possible, take time to talk with your relative and explain your intentions to study and what it will mean to them.
- Where possible involve your relative in the decisions regarding their care.
- Have some 'trial care' days before your course starts and make adjustments where necessary.
- Make an appointment to see your personal tutor and inform them of your additional responsibilities.
- Remember that expert help is available to advise on the care of people with particular conditions. These addresses can be obtained from your local medical practice and the phone book.
- If appropriate, see your relative's general practitioner and discuss the situation with her/him.
- Ensure you leave your contact numbers with all those people who will be involved with the care of your relative: for example, home carer and district nurse.
- If possible approach at least one other person who can be contacted in an emergency.
- A family meeting may be appropriate to discuss the 'new' situation and how other family members can offer help and support.

We are aware that in these situations it is part of one's personal commitment, and although it may be problematic it can be anticipated and arrangements made to adjust your study time. We suggest that students in this position should talk to their personal tutor and inform them of their responsibilities. We also anticipate that the health of both oneself and family members may fluctuate throughout the course; therefore, give some time to think about this and identify how you would cope if this occurred. If carers' leave is required at any time then their tutor will have an understanding of the situation, but communicate this as early as possible and do not leave it until you are desperate.

## Other Dependants?

Looking after dependants is part of life's commitments.
Plan ahead of, and around, the difficulties.
Get help.

## Paid Employment

The authors recognise that students studying nursing do so in one of two ways. First, they may be studying part-time as full-time qualified nurses, in conjunction with their professional job or, second, they may be studying full-time and engaging in additional part-time work to top up their student bursaries. We appreciate that many students struggle financially and take on extra work to support their family commitments, studies or to help pay off their student debts. This frequently involves working as care assistants in hospital settings or nursing homes, in addition to undertaking their study and their clinical placements.

## Learning Aid

How much paid employment do you need to meet your living expenses?
Have you claimed for the benefits you are entitled to?
If you are unsure of your entitlements seek help from the local Social Security Office.

Although understandable, it is our experience that students sometimes get caught up in an ever-decreasing circle, where they need to work in order to stay on the course. They also find that there is little time left to study and, when they do, they are frequently too tired.

We suggest that students take time to work out their expenditure and how much paid work has to be undertaken. The answer must be a compromise and we advise students to reduce their paid employment as much as they can whilst they prepare for assignments and examinations.

## Learning Aid

Student nurses frequently feel exhausted and do not submit work on time when they engage in long and frequent episodes of paid employment.

Beware of becoming entrapped in the work cycle.

Do not compromise on your study.

Balance the budget and studying.

## Students from the UK and Abroad Living on Their Own

We have spent some considerable time discussing the challenges of students who live within busy family households with their many and varied responsibilities. We now consider the challenges faced by students who live alone. The majority (but not all) students are people who are in their late teens and early twenties, who may be living away from home for the first time.

|  | Day | | | | | | |
|---|---|---|---|---|---|---|---|
| **Time** | Mon | Tue | Wed | Thu | Fri | Sat | Sun |
| Early Morning | | | | | | | |
| Mid-morning | | | | | | | |
| Lunch | | | | | | | |
| Early Afternoon | | | | | | | |
| Mid-afternoon | | | | | | | |
| Dinner/Tea | | | | | | | |
| Early Evening | | | | | | | |
| Mid-evening | | | | | | | |
| Late Evening | | | | | | | |
| Notes | | | | | | | |

**Illustration 2:4    Study Plan**

It is our experience that students who live on their own are faced with a number of challenges and these can be summarised as follows:

- Loneliness.
- Boredom.
- Coping with housekeeping details.
- Organising study time.
- Studying alone.

Within this group there are a number of students who have come to study nursing in the UK from abroad. We appreciate that these students have the same anxieties as their colleagues but also have additional issues to deal with; these may include:

- Change of culture: different customs and language difficulties.
- Coping without their family.
- Not communicating with their family for long periods of time.
- Overcoming prejudice of difference.

Fortunately, most people settle into their new student lives well. We suggest that you join some student societies and meet new people, where you can also keep up the hobbies and skills that you have always enjoyed. If you do feel that you are not coping alone, then remember the substantial support that may be offered to you. This might include, first, your fellow students, and you may choose to flat-share if you have been living alone in a bed-sit. Second, your personal tutor will listen and can offer practical help in terms of difficulties with studying or meeting new friends. Finally, the student support department provides a wide range of help including financial advice and support to those with special needs. They also give advice to students who are having difficulties with their particular school or department, which do not appear to be resolved – thankfully this is rare. One of the important things about being a student living alone is that for the first time you may consider yourself to be in a more vulnerable position than previously experienced, and more responsible for your everyday needs. It is at such times that you may reach the decisions that are likely to influence your professional and perhaps personal future, whether this is to work abroad or to pursue studying or to form meaningful relationships.

## Study Time

The above sections discuss how students manage the particular domains in their life to circumscribe study time. The first question that students frequently ask themselves is, 'When can I study?' We answer this question in the manner that readers will now, hopefully, be familiar with–that is with anticipation and forward planning. We ask readers to copy Illustration 2:4 on a sheet of A4 paper and pin it up on a wall where all family members can see it. It is a weekly study-time diary, which students should begin to fill in as soon as they can, and you can pin up four in advance to show a monthly programme. Off-duty, regular family commitments can be included in advance and it can act as a type of calendar. Students can also include assignment deadlines and examination dates, college days and clinical days, and it can also include holidays and reward days so that children can see that they are going to get something in return.

## Learning Aid

Have I copied all my (and family) commitments from my diary onto my study plan(s)? No? Do it now.

Students may choose to study within the formal setting of a college or within the home, where informal study is pursued for assignments and examinations. Some students will find it easier to do most of their study within the college library, perhaps in a group, whilst others will study almost exclusively at home alone. A theme throughout this chapter has been the importance of encouraging students to demonstrate their consideration for others whilst achieving their own goal, and we ask them to be sensitive to the needs of others when creating a study place within the home. We suggest that students confer with the members of their household in deciding where the study place should be and we are aware that for some people space is at a premium. Take time to ask others in the house where a space could be found and involve them in the decision wherever possible. If they think it is their idea they are more likely to give you space and time to study than if you make unilateral decisions. We also know from our own students that finding a quiet place and time to study in a household of noisy flatmates or young children can be very challenging, so lounges and kitchens do not usually make particularly good places to study. It is preferable if you have a space that you can decorate with notes, comments, key facts, acronyms, and so on, which are written on Post-its and stuck on the walls. A space of your own is also preferable if you wish to listen to music whilst studying. It is said that certain music, such as the Baroque composers or Mozart, increases concentration. Box 2:4 provides students with some practical suggestions on finding a space to study.

## Box 2:4   Finding Study Space within the Home

- Agree a suitable study area within the home.
- The study area should be warm and quiet.
- A table where books and work can be left undisturbed is okay, but a room is better.
- An effective light is essential and, where possible, access to natural light is beneficial.
- Space to keep books and files is needed.
- Access to a computer and printer is desirable.
- A dictionary and thesaurus are essential.

## Time to Study?

You are the best person to assess your study needs.

You can study alone or with others.

Talk to family members about study time.

## Leisure Time

We, personally, have experience of how studying can obliterate leisure time as if it never existed at all! Managing time effectively is not about how to fit in slots for studying into a hectic life of responsibilities. It is about achieving a fulfilling life where our needs of work, rest and play are met. Leisure activities are frequently the first to go, and, although understandable, we believe that students should view leisure with the same fervour as they do their other activities; but remember, the priority of the course is to study in order to pass it. Sport and other social recreations serve to relax, keep us fit and give us an opportunity to socialise and learn new skills. All of these pursuits help us to develop our communication, which is a vital requirement of all nurses. In addition we need to spend leisure time with our friends, partners and families to help strengthen these relationships, working towards a 'rounded' and fulfilled lifestyle.

## Time to Play?

Study and work can take over your life.

Balance with leisure.

Plan with others.

Students frequently omit leisure activities from their own study plan. Remember the significance of leisure in achieving a 'rounded' lifestyle.

## Rest and Sleep

We appreciate that rest and sleep do not always come easily. Sleep deprivation not only affects performance but can also have a detrimental effect on physical and mental health. Taking breaks is an important part of planned work, whether it be studying or gardening, and it is better to have frequent short breaks rather than waiting for exhaustion to set in before resting. We suggest that students consider Box 2:5 to help them establish good patterns of sleep and rest.

## Box 2:5    Practical Tips for Rest and Sleep

- Work towards your sleeping area being warm and quiet.
- If you have a baby or dependent relative who requires attention during the night, try and rest or sleep at additional times.
- Do not take studying to bed.
- Your bed should be a place for sleep and relaxation.
- Always ensure you have a period of rest before you go to bed.
- Allowing your mind to 'switch off' after your studying will help relax you.
- Have a milky drink and avoid caffeine drinks before you go to bed – they will only keep you awake.
- Reading non-academic material before you sleep is a good way to relax.
- Take time to organise all that you and your dependants need for the following day. This will ease your mind and help you sleep more easily.

## Responsibilities Towards Other People

As the authors of this text, we have completed all our studies in higher education whilst having extensive responsibilities towards other people, both at home and at work. We know that in the 'world' of nursing studies, the 'ivory tower' rarely exists and that most students do not live in isolation but with other people. Many of these people, as we mention above, are the sole carers for their dependants, and much of this book is concerned with how we navigate our lives to find the time to study. For many students the volume of responsibilities that they have accumulated over the years is large. We recognise that students frequently depend upon the goodwill of others to help them with their responsibilities. For example, the majority of working parents do need a number of reliable friends and family whom they can ask without fear of embarrassment to help out in times of emergency. This act of goodwill, we suggest, should be a two-way process where the neighbourliness is returned.

## Learning Aid

Identify a list of friends and relatives who you can ask to do a favour in relation to childcare, shopping, offering a lift and so on.

Managing time effectively is a skill that is dependent upon anticipating, planning and communicating with others in a considerate and effective way.

## Time for Others?

Others are important.
Relationships should be two-way.
Plan and communicate with significant others.

## Conclusions

We remind students that the skill of managing time effectively is to follow a six-fold plan. First, communicating with family, partners and friends is essential. Discussing courses, study plans, anxieties and addressing the needs of others whilst fulfilling personal goals is the essential first step to successful time management. Second, anticipating the study challenges that lie ahead in terms of the home and work will help in planning the future. Third, planning is crucial whenever there are a lot of issues and a lot of people to consider. Students may find that they can have short-term plans, for example on a weekly basis, and longer-term plans such as for holidays and hospital appointments. Fourth, implementing the original plans in the ways that have been discussed within the home is an important consideration. Fifth, evaluating the plans both individually and collectively with those people who are significant to the student is vital to good communication and 'getting others on your side'. Finally, respond to evaluations by making amendments where necessary.

We conclude this chapter by reassuring students that plans do, sometimes, go wrong and that they should not be disheartened when this happens. Students may add their own suggestions to those that we have provided to embrace their own personal needs, and they may adapt our suggestions wherever necessary to fit their own objectives. We are aware that the demands placed upon our lives change over time and life events carry on regardless of our course of study. Managing time effectively is a skill that is continually being developed and one which we are all engaged in, whatever our position. The secret of time management is to plan it.

---

### SUMMARY POINTS OF CHAPTER 2

- There should be a balance between personal and professional activities, achieving a 'rounded' lifestyle.
- There are special issues relating to those students who study nursing.
- There are serious financial implications for some who study nursing.
- Managing study time within a busy household requires a structured and negotiated approach.
- Responsibilities towards others is important whilst engaging in a programme of study.

## Test Your Study Skills ...

1. What are the issues to consider when organising your study plan? (see page 33)

2. What factors must you anticipate when planning your assignments and examinations? (see page 24)

3. What are the unique challenges faced by students of nursing and how may these be addressed? (see pages 21–23)

4. What features must you consider when prioritising your work? (see page 24)

5. What factors must you consider when organising care for dependent relatives? (see page 28–29)

## Practical Session ...

1. Where appropriate hold a meeting with partner/family to discuss study time within the household.

2. Produce a personal plan identifying all commitments to family and work.

3. Highlight the proposed study time on the above personal plan.

4. Identify support networks to help with family commitments.

5. Identify support systems within the college.

6. Adopt the habit of keeping a diary.

7. If you have a dependent relative, keep a file with relevant information, including telephone numbers and details of groups and organisations who may offer help and support.

# 3 Technology for Nurses

**LEARNING OUTCOMES**

1. To understand the importance of technology for nurses.
2. To be aware of practical tasks to overcome the fear of computers.
3. To be able to get started with a word-processing program.
4. To be familiar with the basic terminology of computer language.
5. To appreciate the growing areas in which IT is important for nurses.

## Introduction

This chapter will outline the growth in information technology (IT), particularly in relation to healthcare settings. For many this explosion in IT has created an element of fear or anxiety regarding the use of computers and this will be discussed in terms of employing a mature response and avoiding the fear. At the very least, the majority of nurses will be expected to be able to use a word-processing package and we will outline the basics of getting started with this; with the huge amount of information created in healthcare settings it is not surprising that technology is now employed to manage this. Therefore, there is now a close relationship between IT and learning, and we will discuss the importance of this in contemporary study.

## What is Information Technology?

Simply stated, IT refers to how knowledge, facts, figures and material are managed, sorted, stored, moved around and accessed by others. Before the printing press, information was passed on from one generation to another by word of mouth or on handwritten parchments. However, once printing was developed, it revolutionised how information could be managed, stored and accessed by successive generations. Think of your college library and the rows of shelves with their books and journals; this has been the method of storage for hundreds of years. Now the information that is contained in the books and journals can be stored on computer and may one day replace them (many books and journals are now available electronically). Computers come in all shapes and sizes and were originally designed to compute mathematical figures and were extremely large and cumbersome. However, they now come as palm-tops (to fit in the palm of your hand), hand-held (slightly larger than palm), lap-tops (to sit on your lap), personal computers (PCs, to sit on your desk) and supercomputers that are used in major science laboratories and universities around the world. There is little point in listing all the many and varied types of computers, as by the time these words are in print the market will have changed significantly with the constant developments in technology. However, what we can do is to identify the basic components of a computer system.

## Unsure of the 'Language' of Technology?

Computers come in many shapes and sizes.
Hardware refers to the physical items.
Software refers to the programs.
The 'language' can be offputting.

The first distinction to be drawn in computer terminology is between the *hardware* and the *software*. The hardware refers to the computer itself, the drive, monitor (screen), keyboard, speakers, printers, mouse, boards and chips. They are the items that have a physical presence and you can feel and touch them. Software, on the other hand, is concerned with the programs, sometimes called applications, which are written for the computer and are of two types. The first are programs that make the computer work, and the second are the programs that manage information of one description or another. They include statistical packages, word-processing programs, spreadsheets, graphics, games and the many, many programs that manufacturers make. This knowledge of the hardware and software is sufficient to get you going if you are new to computers. However, IT and computer language is foreign to many and you may wish to refer to Appendix 1 for some basic definitions of this new terminology.

The world of information technology employs a discourse that many of us may not be too familiar with, but as with all foreign languages the more we understand what the words mean, and the more we use them, the more familiar we will become. We often hear the word 'bytes' used when discussing computers, which simply refers to the extent of memory that the computer has. However, there is often confusion as to what this means when it is used as a suffix with other words. Box 3:1 gives us an indication as to what these 'byte terms' mean.

## Box 3:1    The Byte System (adapted from Thede, 1999)

| Byte Name | Number of Bytes |
| --- | --- |
| Kilobyte | 1,024 |
| Megabyte | 1,048,576 |
| Gigabyte | 1,073,741,824 |
| Terabyte | 1,099,511,627,776 |
| Petabyte | 1,125,899,906,842,624 |
| Exabyte | 1,152,921,504,606,846,976 |
| Zettabyte | 1,000,000,000,000,000,000,000 (approximately) |
| Yottabyte | 1,000,000,000,000,000,000,000,000 (approximately) |

## Overcoming Fear of Computers

Fear of IT and computers is likely to be based either on unfamiliarity with them or a bad experience of them. In either event you will probably think that they look complicated and are very technical and require great skill and expertise to make them work effectively. They may look very fragile to you and you may think that they are easily broken. Many people believe that they will do damage to the equipment and press all the wrong buttons, which will break the system. They are fearful that any mistakes cannot be rectified and that they are bound to erase information from the storage system. They are worried that they are slow and do not know how to proceed through a program. They are anxious that they do not know what to look at on the screen or look for on the keyboard. Some people are afraid that their lack of computer and IT knowledge will make them look foolish and some are ashamed that they cannot even turn a computer on.

## Learning Aid

What are your main fears regarding IT and computers?

All these fears and concerns are real to you and are, therefore, to be taken seriously. However, the vast majority of them are groundless and you can overcome the anxieties through a series of strategies. The first approach is to recognise the avoidance strategies that you adopt to steer clear of computers. This might include getting others to do the work for you, rationalising that you can manage without it, believing that your work is of sufficient quality without it, and putting it off until another day. Whatever your avoidance strategies are, reveal them to yourself and recognise them for what they are. Make yourself find a computer that is switched off and touch it, press all the keys on the keyboard, pretend that you are an expert typist and press the keys as if you were typing. Of course, as the computer is switched off, nothing will happen, but as a starting point this will help you overcome your fear of it.

## Learning Aid

Learn how to use a spreadsheet, word-processing package and a
graphics program at a basic level. Play with old equipment and documents.
Fear will be overcome by familiarity.
Seek help and do not avoid addressing the fear.

There are many external courses that you can attend to help you, either as a newcomer or at advanced levels, and many universities and colleges run their own internal courses either through IT departments or libraries. Find out what is available and choose the ones most appropriate to your needs. We will outline the basics of a word-processing package in the next section as this is likely to be your main requirement for writing assignments and projects for your course.

## Word-processing

Most universities and colleges now request that essays, assignments, literature reviews, and so on, be submitted in a word-processed format. This is due to the easy accessibility to computers for most people in contemporary times, and even though a particular individual may not possess their own computer they are likely to be able to access one in a library or college department. Although you can still obtain machines that do word-processing only, most PCs are purchased with a word-processor as part of a package of programs, including spreadsheets, graphics, and so on. We will outline Microsoft Word™ as it is the most commonly used word-processor. Word-processors allow you to type up your work, save it on the hard drive (and back it up on a memory stick or a removable disk) and then to re-visit it as many times as you like to edit it, add to it or subtract from it.

We strongly recommend that you write your project or assignment in longhand, either in pencil or pen, before typing it into your word-processor. It may feel tempting to sit down at a computer screen and type directly into the computer, believing that you are saving yourself some time. However, in our experience, there are few students

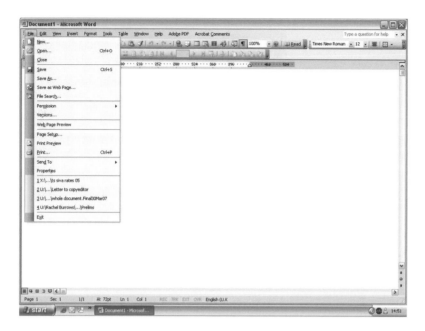

**Screen shot of Microsoft Word used by permission of Microsoft Corporation**

(or lecturers) who can do this successfully and achieve a sufficiently high-quality standard of writing. We suggest that you read Chapter 5 on writing assignments and make sure that you plan thoroughly and write out your work before typing it in to the computer. This will give you a chance to edit your work when typing up.

## Learning Aid

Word-processor programs do not replace 'thinking'. Computers compute but they cannot 'think'.

Let us now briefly work through the basics of constructing a typed version of your project. In most word-processor programs you have an open document to work on as you go into the program, but if not then you can open a new document by clicking on the 'File' drop-down menu button at the top left position and choosing 'New'.

The screen will usually show two bars of options at the top of the screen: (a) a series of words which are called drop-down menus, such as 'File', 'Edit', 'Insert', and so on, and (b) a bar of small icons below the words. If you click on the drop-down menus you will be offered a series of further choices to make, and the icons on the second bar refer to one specific function only. There are usually two rulers to be seen: one at the top between the page and the icons and one at the left between the page and the edge of the computer. At the bottom of the screen there is the status line, between the 'Drawing' icon bar and the 'Start' functions, which tells you where you are in the document and what functions you have switched on: for example, 'Caps Lock' for capital letters.

## Want to Word-process?

Most commonly used programs for students.
May be mandatory for some courses.

## Typing in your text

There are basically two modes of typing in your words. The first is where you merely type in new text on to the blank screen, whilst the second refers to where you type in new text over old unwanted text. In this latter mode you need to press the key 'Insert' on the keyboard and this function is called 'Typeover' or 'Overwrite'; when switched on this will be indicated in the status line. However, we do not recommend the latter as the 'Insert' key can be a dangerous beast!

## Learning Aid

Often the 'Insert' key is pressed inadvertently and when you are inserting in new text you overwrite what you have previously written, thus losing your original words. Beware!

## Learning Aid

Learn to type properly at a basic level. This can be done in two weeks, undertaking 30 minutes' practice per day. There are books on the market as well as open learning courses, evening courses and professional instruction available. (Irecently receivedthefirste-mailfrommy89yearoldmotherwhocouldn'tfindthespacebar!)

## Blocking text

You may wish to delete, move, copy or change the style and size of your text that you have already typed in. You can do this, as well as many other functions, by 'blocking' the text you wish to work on or change in some way. 'Blocking' is done by putting the cursor at the beginning (or end) of the required text, clicking and holding the mouse's left button and dragging the cursor on the screen to the end of the required text (or beginning). It will change colour to highlight which text has been 'blocked', and you then release the mouse button. You are then ready to do your changes (delete, copy, cut, etc.). There are other ways of 'blocking' text, but this is sufficient to get started, and please note that we have assumed that you are using a mouse. Many of these procedures can be undertaken on the keyboard by the use of the arrow keys in conjunction with the shift key.

## Learning Aid

A line can be 'blocked' by moving the cursor to the left of the line until it changes into an arrow and then clicking.

A sentence can be 'blocked' by holding down the CTRL key and then clicking anywhere in the sentence.

A paragraph can be 'blocked' by moving the cursor to the left of the paragraph until it changes to an arrow and then double-clicking. Or triple-click anywhere in the paragraph.

## Fonts and sizes

In the icon bar at the top of the screen you will see the type of letter style (font) that the computer is set to use and next to it the size of letter being typed. These are known as default settings, which are set originally by the manufacturer and remain the same when the computer is switched off, but which you can change if you wish. You can change both the font style and size of text by clicking on the arrow next to where it indicates the font and choosing one of the style options available. This can also be done with the size of the text next to it. Box 3:2 shows a few of the more common fonts and sizes that are used.

## Box 3:2   Some Font Styles and Sizes

This is Book Antiqua with font size 8

This is Berlin with font size 10

This is Times New Roman with font size 12

This is Garamond with font size 12

## THIS IS ALGERIAN WITH FONT SIZE 14

*(Continued)*

*(Continued)*

This is Arial with font size 14

This is Berlin Sans FB with font size 16

# This is Broadway with font size 20

(This is the one that my 13-year-old daughter uses to try and convince the teacher that she has written a lot – it doesn't work, as currently the teacher is smarter than my 13-year-old!)

## Emphasis

You can produce emphasis by using bold, italics and underlining (in any combination). These buttons are usually at the top of the screen towards the right and are indicated by their initial letter and their style (B, *I*, <u>U</u>). Simply click on them when they are required and again to turn them off.

## Margins

The word-processing program will set the default setting for the margins but you can change them if you wish. You can do this by clicking on the small arrows in the rulers and dragging them to your required position. The top ruler governs the left and right margins of the page whilst the left ruler governs the top and bottom margins.

## Learning Aid

The margin settings can be a little tricky for the newcomer, so the novice may wish to leave the margins as set.

## Deleting Text

There are three main ways of deleting text. First, go to the beginning of the unwanted text and press down the 'Delete' key once and this will remove one character to the right of the cursor; if you hold the key down it will speed up and begin to remove characters faster. Second, you can go to the end of the unwanted text and then press down the 'Backspace' key (top right of the main keys in the keyboard, indicated by a left pointing arrow). Press once for one character or hold down to speed up. This will remove characters to the left of the cursor. Third, you can 'block' the unwanted text as indicated above and then press 'Delete' or 'Backspace' once.

## Cutting, Copying and Moving Text

You can undertake these operations by 'blocking' the required text, clicking on the 'Edit' drop-down menu button at the top of the screen and selecting 'Cut' if you want to delete it or move it, or 'Copy' if you want to duplicate the text somewhere else in your document. Then, move the cursor to the position where you want to place the 'Cut' text or 'Copied' text, select the 'Edit' drop-down menu, and select 'Paste'. This will place the text in the document forwards from where you placed the cursor.

## Page Numbers

Page numbers are easily inserted by clicking on the 'Insert' drop-down menu button at the top of the screen and clicking on 'Page Numbers'. You will be asked where you want the page numbers to be placed on your pages and you will be given a number of options. Choose accordingly and then press 'OK'.

## Justification

This refers to the text on the page being set in one of four ways. 'Left Justification' is where the words on the page are flush with the left margin. 'Right Justification' is where the text is flush with the right margin. 'Centre Justification' refers to each line being centred between the margins and 'Full Justification' is where the text is flush with both left and right margins. The buttons for this are usually at the top of the screen to the right, and show a series of little lines to represent text on a page. Merely click on the required button.

## Saving

Obviously, saving your work is a very important function, and one that should be done very regularly as you are working on your document. When typing on to the screen we would recommend saving every few sentences, and if formatting your document with 'Bold', 'Italics' or 'Underline' we would recommend saving after each page has been completed.

## Learning Aid

If you lose power to your computer or it ceases to respond for any reason (see 'Crashes ...' below) you will lose any work that you have done since your last save. So, save frequently.

Saving can be done by clicking on the 'File' drop-down menu button and choosing 'Save' or 'Save As'. This latter function allows you to name the file and tell the computer where you want it saved to. Your file can be saved to a number of sources. It can be saved to the hard drive within your computer itself, usually referred to as the local 'C' drive. It can be saved to a 'floppy disk' (which actually is not floppy) referred to as a 3½" floppy 'A' drive. The floppy disk is usually inserted into a slot in the front of the computer. This can then be removed and transported to another computer. Unfortunately, there is not much memory on floppies to save vast amounts of data. Fortunately, however technology has advanced and there are now available various 'memory sticks' which can hold large amounts of information. Various firms now produce removable disks which are inserted in other drives of the computer usually referred to by another letter of the alphabet. There are also memory sticks that are inserted in USB ports, which are small oblong port-hole connections in the computer. You may also be able to save your file to a CD in drive 'D' but unlike the other means this is usually a fixed save and you cannot work on the file with repeated savings. This type of save is known as being 'burnt' on the disk.

## Learning Aid

Take time to look at a computer (not the screen) and check how many drives (slots) and USBs (small oblong port-holes) there are in it. Check for lids and buttons that open the drives.

## Printing

Once you are satisfied with your document, you can print it and read it for editing. Click on the 'File' drop-down menu button and click print. You will then be asked whether you want to print the entire document, the current page (where the cursor is placed), or a number of pages (for example, 4–6). Click on the required option and then click 'OK'.

## Track Changes

Another feature of word-processing that is being more commonly used is that of 'track changes'. Although it is fair to say that it is largely the publishing houses that are more commonly employing track changes when editing manuscripts for publication, it is also increasingly being used for students submitting drafts of work for lecturers. Its main features are that, when editing or changing a text, the material that is altered does not disappear but instead goes into a 'balloon' at the right margin. The new inserted material appears in a different colour so that the reader can easily see what has been removed and what has been inserted. There are usually three types of balloons; formatted, comment and deleted. These are self-explanatory, in that they highlight changes in format, any comments or queries and the deleted material. The location of track changes is in the 'Tools' drop-down menu and you merely click on track changes. An icon will appear in the top toolbar and TRK will be highlighted in the status bar at the bottom. To turn track changes off merely click on the icon in the top toolbar and TRK will be dimmed in the status bar, indicating it is turned off.

## Crashes, Hang-Ups and Freezes

Even when you have done everything correctly and you are proficient with computer technology, problems can still occur. Sometimes the computer ceases to respond to your commands and no matter what you do it will not proceed. This is called by numerous names: the ones we are able to repeat are crashes, hang-ups and freezes! In this event wait a few minutes to see if it clears and if not then press 'CTRL', 'ALT' and 'DELETE' at the same time. Your computer will shut down and then restart itself again. You will lose any work that you have done up to the last time that you 'Saved' your work. Therefore, we reiterate, save regularly.

If 'CTRL', 'ALT' and 'DELETE' does not respond you may need to press the restart button on your computer or turn the power off and then on again to restart it. Again, you will lose the work since the last 'Saved' and you may, rarely, lose some saved information on certain files.

## Learning Aid

Some people cause 'crashes' by overloading the computer with operations by pressing the keys before previous operations have been completed. Patience is a virtue.

## Learning Aid

What is your main concern regarding having a go with a word-processing package? If it is worry about making mistakes then read the section on 'Fear and Confidence' in this chapter again. Borrow from someone an old unwanted document that is saved on a removable disk. Save it to a hard drive under your own title and practise the above operations. It will not matter if mistakes are made as it will remain unchanged on the removable disk.

# Other Common Programs

There are lots of programs that can be used on computers, from many different companies. However, we will restrict ourselves to the two most commonly used programs from Microsoft.

## Excel

Microsoft Excel is a spreadsheet program that is capable of calculation and producing graphics for display. A spreadsheet is basically constituted of rows and columns of individual cells in which data is put. The data can be numbers and therefore subject to numerical manipulation, for example with statistics, or it can be letters and hold written information. Once data is put into Excel it can produce an array of visual displays such as pie-charts, bar-charts, etc.

## Powerpoint

This is another very popular Microsoft program and is increasingly being used in the classroom setting by lecturing and teaching staff. It is a presentation program which is used by business people, educators and trainers in a wide variety of settings. Powerpoint is a series of slides that can take various formats, with a huge number of background colours and illustrations. The slides can be animated in a variety of ways with the words zooming in from a particular direction or crystallizing in some way. The visual display can be extremely entertaining. However, herein lies one of the criticisms

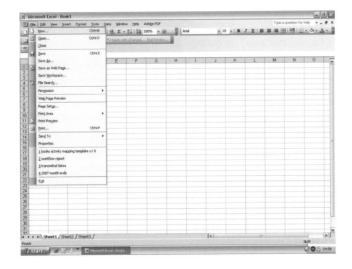

**Screen shot of Microsoft Excel used by permission of Microsoft Corporation**

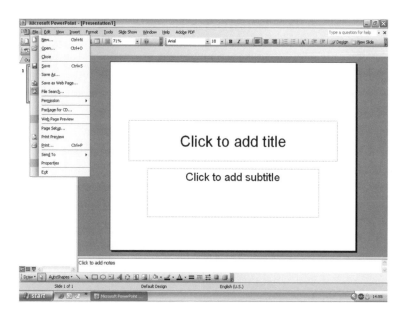

**Screen shot of Microsoft PowerPoint used by permission of Microsoft Corporation**

of it, namely the distinction between form and content. A lively, entertaining and animated presentation may have poor content, and vice versa. The former is known as 'Death by Powerpoint'.

## Interactive Whiteboards

An interactive whiteboard is an electronic writing surface that captures notes, usually on computer, when written on the board, though some newer models have an electronic functionality within the board itself. Interactive whiteboards are used for group sessions, usually the classroom, and can be connected to web-sites or software programmes such as Powerpoint presentations.

## Learning Aid

In the list of programs, open up Excel and type in numbers in a few cells in both rows and columns, and click on the graphics at the top. See how many displays you can create.

Open up Powerpoint and try to create a fictitious presentation (tip – new slides are in the insert drop-down menu).

# Learning and Technology

The psychology of learning teaches us that if we have a desire to learn something then we are more likely to learn it than if we did not have that desire. At first this appears to be an obvious statement. However, we only need to ask ourselves why it is that we have not learnt something that we have had a desire to learn (i.e. to play a musical instrument or to learn a foreign language). It would seem that merely having a desire to learn something is not enough in itself. We need to ask ourselves how strong that desire is or where the desire is ranked amongst all the other things that we wish to do in life. Thus, learning seems dependent on a number of interrelated factors. First, there is a relationship between learning a practical skill, such as managing a computer, and the cognitive skills of knowing and memorising information effectively. This is important to us if we are to overcome our anxieties of learning new technology or managing computers satisfactorily. We may need to work our way carefully through manuals, guides and step-by-step practice sheets, but this is only a first stage until we retain the information and are able to recall it when required. Only through the process of practice, trial and error and learning through reflection will we acquire the balance between a practice skill and a cognitive skill. It is very much the same when we learn to drive a car and at first find it difficult to co-ordinate all the individual skills to get from A to B. Once these skills are acquired most journeys do not phase us, although good and bad drivers continue to exist!

## Learning Technology?

Learn to learn.
Practise learning.
Know your technology well.

Second, learning is also concerned with acquiring facts, figures and knowledge in general about a particular topic that can be used in practice whenever necessary. For example, we may not need to know the intricate details of, say, computer programming, but some fundamental information is helpful to us in using computers at a basic level. Third, learning is also concerned with making sense of the information that we receive, formulating meaning from it and relating it to everyday life. We can see the importance of this for us in the advancement of information technology in healthcare practice, and only if we can make sense of this will we be able to overcome our fear and ignorance. When the technology and computer equipment have a direct relevance to us in the clinical, educational or research setting then we will be in a stronger position in terms of our confidence to address them. Fourth, learning is also about understanding the world through constantly reinterpreting the knowledge that we have about it. This makes our world, and in our case the healthcare setting, a fluid dynamic state and not a static and fixed entity. We must reinterpret the practice area in which we work and reformulate interpretations that construct our knowledge.

## Learning Aid

What everyday practical uses could you make of a computer, for example writing letters, making lists, compiling a telephone and address book, using the calculator, playing games, etc.?

# Technology and Some of its Uses for Nurses

Finally in this chapter, we will outline a few of the uses that technology has for those in the healthcare arena in relation to learning, communication, theorising and recording patient care. The first to be dealt with are learning uses.

## Learning Uses

Computerised assisted learning (CAL) programs are becoming increasingly available in many fields of study, and health-related courses are now available in topics relevant to medicine and nursing. Most programs are interactive; that is, they request that you do something, tell you whether you have made the right response, and, if you have answered correctly, will ask you to do a further task. A CAL program is a good teacher, in that it can make you work over a problem until you make the right response, set you tasks on your weaker aspects, reiterate important issues, is extremely patient and is always attentive. However, as a teacher a CAL program has its downside. They can be very pedantic and will not let you progress until you have mastered what they want you to learn. They can be limited in not really knowing whether you 'know' something or why it is that you cannot learn a particular point. They can also make you feel controlled and they can become frustrating. Notwithstanding these limitations, if the programs are written well they can be a valuable way of learning, depending on the individuality of each and every student.

The second major computerised learning utility is the Internet. Few will not have heard of the Internet, even though many may not have had the opportunity to use it, and some may even have avoided it like the plague. Simply stated, the Internet represents a vast computer network, which can put you in touch with a massive source of information, on an almost limitless number of topics, from all over the world. It does not exist in itself as a single site but is connected by people and computers via cables, wires and telephone lines. All you need is a computer, a modem and a telephone line connection. Anyone can put information on the Internet, both individuals and organisations. However, this does raise questions as to how reliable the information actually is on the Internet and you need to check your sources very carefully before relying upon it. Some books are available electronically, which you can download for your personal use on your computer screen. Although one may not wish to read an entire book on screen you may like to read a short section or even a chapter via this method. There are also formal data banks placed on the Internet by reputable organisations and institutions, which can be used for research purposes. However, for all these sources of information take great care that you do not break copyright rules. You may use quotes as you would in a book, of course, but ensure that you reference the source accordingly and conform to the rules regarding appropriate referencing styles (see Chapter 6).

## Learning Aid

There is a large amount of information on the Internet that is relevant to healthcare professionals. However, do not rely solely on this as markers look for a good balance of sources.

One final point will be made regarding the Internet and that is its globalisation in relation to both the information that is available and the individuals who can access it. Health-related information is in abundance on the Internet and carries information about particular diseases and illness which is available to both professional students of health, and to sufferers of many conditions. This leads to patients accessing this information and becoming much more informed about their condition, and in some cases even more informed than the professional. This is a good thing in that patients and professionals can work together as a team in trying to help the sufferer. Finally, there are many health-related courses that are now available on the Internet and students of a particular course may now come from all over the world. You may end up on a course where your fellow students come from, say, Australia, New Zealand, Canada, Argentina or America.

## Communication Uses

Communication via technology has never been easier and although some systems are technologically complex their use is simple. The first to be mentioned is the e-mail system. Electronic mail means that if your computer is networked to another computer you can send a message to it, and receive one from it, if connected by a modem. There are basically two types of e-mail: (a) a network connected locally within an organisation such as a university or NHS trust and (b) a global network that is connected by telephone lines. Each person, or site, has a unique e-mail address and you can send messages to single users or to a whole list of people, depending on your choice. There is a facility to attach documents to your message so you can send your projects and assignments through to tutors and lecturers if this is acceptable to them. Remember that this will depend on the recipient having the resources to print out assignments and projects, and if there are a number of students on the course then the resources in computers, printers, print cartridges, paper and time will be considerable for lecturers and tutors.

## Learning Aid

Check list with the recipient, whoever they are, before sending big attachments which will demand a lot of resources to print out.

E-mail communication is a valuable medium but its main drawback is the number of unwanted messages that are received. It needs to be managed in a mature and sensible manner. There is a general code of practice relating to the use of e-mail which is referred to as 'netiquette', and is based on good manners and common sense. There is also a facility on the e-mail to let you know when the message, sent or received, has been opened. Therefore, be careful that you do not say that you have not received a message when it has been indicated that it has been opened – at least by someone.

Personal diaries can also be managed via e-mail and meetings arranged even when the recipient's computer is switched off. There is also a facility to look into other people's diaries and to see if they are available at a particular time, on a particular day (although they cannot necessarily see what you are engaged in when not available). Many people find this intrusive, but remember you do not have to activate this facility if you do not wish to, unless it is an employer requirement.

The second communication use is the multi-media system, which overlaps with the learning uses above to some degree. This is a system that employs a range of communication strategies such as music soundtracks, films, cartoons, graphics, photographic stills, voiceovers and text. These are employed to help the student explore a particular topic in a variety of ways. These educational packages are increasingly available and allow much exploration from screen to screen, as you move through the numerous facilities. They are similar to computer encyclopaedias in which you can click on certain topics and explore the issues.

The third communication use to be mentioned is the computer conferencing system, which is an expansion of the e-mail facility as outlined above. In this, all messages are sent to everyone who is a conference member and everyone can respond by posting their message on a shared computer notice board. Thus, it is an open system that everyone can get involved in and these systems tend to initiate many levels of discussion.

## Communication and Nursing?

E-mail systems.
Personal diaries.
Multi-media systems.
Computer conferencing systems.

## Theorising and recording uses

The third area of use of technology for us in nursing healthcare settings is how it can help theorising about, and recording of, patient care. Computerised modelling is used where information processing is particularly complicated, for example, in showing how weather formations are likely to react, in showing how molecules are formed, what the damage of volcanic reactions, earthquakes and tidal waves is likely to be, and so on. It is used in medical science to model drug reactions, cell processes, organ transplant rejection processes, etc. Modelling can be both pictorial as in moving film, graphs, charts, etc., or may be mathematical as in the production of formulae and complex equations.

## Theorising and Recording Nursing?

Computerised modelling.
Nursing classificatory systems.

Nursing classificatory systems have been developed to assist in patient care delivery. They are computerised attempts to standardise the language of nursing in order for it to be accessible to others in the healthcare team. They are databases that employ structured information to be entered when patient care is delivered and vary in their overall approach. There are sets and sub-sets of information, which can be used to plan further care and communicate what has been undertaken in care delivery. Computerised patient records are now a common feature in most clinical settings and are used to input data on a patient's care. They are designed to be quickly retrieved and linked to other sources of information regarding the patient, so can be used holistically. Thus, it seems that technology is ever-present and encroaching more and more into all aspects of healthcare delivery.

# Conclusions

Many people do not like the advance of technology into every aspect of their lives, including its encroachment into medicine, nursing and healthcare in general. However, it does have huge advantages and can advance patient care considerably, not only in relation to the computerised investigations that can be carried out, or the computer-assisted exploratory surgical techniques, but also in recording patient care with, hopefully, less chance of medical records going missing. In nursing we are faced with the same increase in technology as are many others in the healthcare team. Therefore, we need to overcome any fears that we have of managing the technology and especially the computers. In this chapter we have outlined some ideas and hints for anxious students to overcome their fears and have a go. The best method of overcoming the fear of computers is to find one that you can play with – and enjoy making the mistakes.

---

## SUMMARY POINTS OF CHAPTER 3

- Information technology is here and here to stay.
- There has been a growth in the use of technology in healthcare settings.
- Many people have a fear of computers and there are strategies for overcoming this.
- Most nurses will be called upon to use a word-processing program.
- There is a close relationship between learning and technology.

---

# Test Your Study Skills ...

1. What strategies are available to you to help you to overcome your fear of computers? (see pages 41–42)

2. Name five hardware items and three types of software programs. (see page 40)

3. What is a font? (see pages 45–46)

4. How do you 'block' a piece of text? (see pages 44–45)

5. How does IT assist nurses? (see page 56)

6. What is 'netiquette'? (see page 55)

## Practical Session ...

Access a word-processing program and ...

1. Open a new blank document and save it to a removable disk using your own file name (see page 43).

2. Type in one paragraph about your life in font Garamond, size 14, and save it (see page 45).

3. Emphasise every line using alternate Bold, Italics and Underline. (see page 47). Save it.

4. Delete the middle sentence (see pages 44–45).

5. Save it and print it out (see page 48).

# 4 Managing Literature and Related Material

## LEARNING OUTCOMES

1. To understand the importance and relevance of supporting literature.
2. To be able to access literature from a variety of sources.
3. To be able to produce a literature review for assessed work.
4. To know how to incorporate a literature review within the main body of a text.

## Introduction

With the huge expansion in information regarding healthcare delivery it is of paramount importance to be able to manage this literature. Clearly, we cannot read everything that is written and we must be able to focus more specifically on the available evidence. In this chapter we will emphasise the importance of managing the literature and outline strategies for dealing with this. Reviewing the literature is a central task for nursing students and we will highlight how this is undertaken in relation to acquiring the literature, reading and critiquing it. Practical ways in which the literature can be managed will also be outlined.

## The Need for Managing Literature

The first point that we would like to make concerning the ability to manage literature and related material refers to knowing and managing the *evidence* pertaining to a particular topic. This is not to say, of course, that all literature is good evidence, but merely that all literature, and related material, is evidence of one sort or another. Clearly, as time progresses, with every passing week, more and more literature is being produced, which adds to the ever-increasing amount that we have to manage. We may hope that each and every piece of material that is produced adds to a specific knowledge base and creates a greater focus on specific topics. However, in reality, we know that this is not the case and part of our management skills in relation to the literature concerns the ability to distinguish between the good and the bad, the wheat and the chaff, so to speak.

As the literature grows it is important that each item (article, book, report, etc.) is examined for relevancy and accuracy, and is synthesised into an overall theoretical framework. It may be rejected on the grounds of scientific validity but incorporated as subjective anecdotal evidence.

The second point in establishing the skills of literature management is closely related to the first, but is also a consequence of it. That is, as knowledge has grown it has created the need for specialists to focus on more specific areas of practice. This is well recognised in medicine and surgery with 'experts' emerging in very precise areas of practice. However, it is also occurring in other areas of healthcare practice from radiotherapy to occupational therapy, and from physiotherapy to nursing. In the case of the latter discipline the growth in Nursing and Midwifery Council (NMC) courses, which focus on specialist areas and offer specific qualifications, is an indication of the development of the specialist practitioner programme.

Whilst everyone who undertakes basic general training in their discipline receives a broad knowledge base, the growth in knowledge means that few, if any, can know a great deal about all specialist areas. Thus, managing the growing literature requires specific knowledge, understanding and skills.

## Learning Aid

Know and manage the literature on your topic.

Become a 'specialist' in your area.

Many students have feelings of anxiety, and even panic, at having to work in the library. If you have not received training in managing the library then take courage and ask the librarian for help. It is their job, and they are usually pleased to be of assistance. It is easy to feel overwhelmed by the vast amount of literature that is written for nurses. Do not avoid going in to the library. Spend as much time in there as you can. Confidence in your library skills will help prevent you feeling that you cannot cope.

## Growth of Nursing Literature

Fifty years ago the number of nursing journals that was available to student nurses in the course of their study was in the low single figures. Today, nursing journals alone number in the hundreds. The vast majority have a specialist focus (e.g. *Journal of Diabetes Nursing*), or 'corner' of the nursing market (e.g. *Nurse Education Today*); some are geared towards a local or national market (e.g. *Utah Nurse*) whilst others have an international target (e.g. *International Journal of Nursing Studies*). Some nursing journals are peer-reviewed, that is, articles are sent, anonymised, to specialists in a relevant field, for their appraisal, who may request amendments be undertaken before publication, or may suggest that the article be rejected completely. Other nursing journals are not peer-reviewed and they rely on the editor, or the editorial board, as a review process. However, the peer-review process is considered the 'safer' in terms of producing some degree of academic rigour. It should also be noted that journals, from all disciplines, come and go. Many are brought into existence but fail to survive, or are taken over by another publishing house who may absorb them, re-name them, or re-focus them. However, the literature that has been produced during the course of their existence is just as relevant as the literature that is produced in 'live' journals, and can be referenced in the same manner.

Whilst journals probably account for the major source of information for most nurses, the growth in 'literature' now covers an even wider sphere, particularly in response to the developments in information technology. Box 4:1 highlights just some of the sources of material that can be reviewed and referenced by the discerning nurse.

We can see from this list that there are rich areas to be drawn from in order to provide a comprehensive coverage, a rigorous review and a thorough analysis. However, a note of caution is worthy of mention here. *Primary sources* of literature refer to the original authors who have produced their own work, and their own interpretations, whereas *secondary sources* refer to those authors who interpret others' work. The sources in a table might well be primary sources but may well be of a secondary nature. Therefore, the student should ensure that they cover their primary areas first and use the secondary sources as just that, secondary.

The growth in literature has occurred not only in nursing but also in every other discipline, related or unrelated, to healthcare practice. Just as in the past the student nurse would be referred to books and journals in anatomy, physiology, psychology, sociology, social work, public health, and so on, the same is the case today. Therefore, this means that the nurse currently engaged in managing the literature has the greatest wealth of material to cover, and more than any other previous nursing group. See Illustration 4:1.

## Learning Aid

The 'literature' comes from a wide variety of sources.
It is constantly expanding.
Journals account for the major source.
Use primary sources first, then secondary sources.

## Box 4:1    Some Sources of 'Literature'

| Sources | Example |
| --- | --- |
| Abstracts | Summary works |
| Artistic works | Poetry |
| Audio-visual material | Documentaries |
| Book, chapters | Specific chapter(s) within book |
| Book, whole | Whole book covers the topic |
| Case reports | Inquiries |
| Computer programs | Numerous aids to research |
| Conference proceedings | Keynote speeches, concurrent sessions, posters |
| Electronic databases | Growing number available for researchers |
| Hearings | Inquests, judicial reviews, case hearings |
| Internet | www |
| Journals | *Journal of Advanced Nursing* |
| Magazines | *Cheshire Life* |
| Motion pictures | *The English Patient* |
| Newspapers | *Guardian* |
| Pamphlets | *Pro Life* |
| Personal communications | Letters to editors |
| Reports | The Beverly Allitt Inquiry |
| Serials | Books, monographs |
| Theses/dissertations | MSc, MA, MPhil, PhD |
| Unpublished works | Reports, studies, correspondences |

However, as we can see, they do not have as much to cover as the nurses of next year will have, as they will have another year's production to review.

Another growth area is much more of a help than a hindrance and that is the increased focus on evidence-based practice. This means that we can concentrate on literature and related material that produces empirical evidence. In its widest sense this refers to information that is derived from experience of the external world, rather than from internal speculation. However, to avoid a complex philosophical discussion we can narrow this to literature that is research based. Although research can fall into any number of categories, with each one having a degree of scientific 'weight', depending on professional discipline, a framework that is often used follows that outlined in Box 4:2.

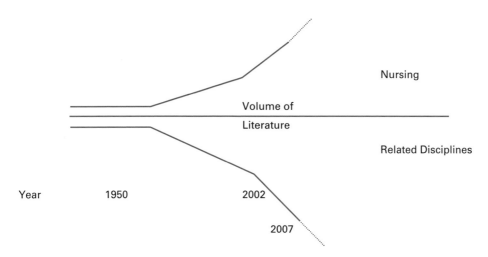

Nursing

Volume of

Literature

Related Disciplines

Year                    1950                    2002

                                        2007

**Illustration 4.1    Growing volume of literature**

## Learning Aid

Learn how to undertake a systematic review of the literature and be able
to distinguish between this and a meta-analysis.

With the growth in literature in many fields of healthcare, as we mentioned above, it
may not be feasible to read everything that has been published on a particular topic.
Furthermore, even where it has been possible to read all the material, the diversity
of the quality of publications may make its synthesis problematic. Thus, systematic
reviews have been developed to overcome this difficulty. Box 4:2 shows a research
design framework in which published articles can be evaluated and located in one of the
five categories. They are categorised with a weighting of 1 to 5, which represents an
assessment of scientific evidence, in relation to the effectiveness of an intervention in a
specific healthcare area. At the top of the hierarchy there are experimental studies,
which are rated as having significant 'scientific' rigour and include randomised control
trials. At the bottom of the hierarchy there is 'scientific' evidence based on expert opinion. In between these two poles there are graded 'scientific' approaches. In medicine the
main focus is upon the randomised control trials, and if enough of these types of studies exist then they are usually relied upon to form medical opinion on whether an intervention is appropriate or not. However, in nursing few randomised controls of nursing
interventions actually exist and therefore other levels of 'scientific' evidence are usually
incorporated into the overall developmental theory.

## Box 4:2    Research Design Framework (adapted from NHS CRD, 2001)

| Research Design | Example/Type |
| --- | --- |
| 1. Experimental Studies | Studies in which variables are controlled and some conditions are randomised, i.e. allocation of subjects into experimental groups with full concealment. |
| 2. Quasi-experimental Studies | Studies in which the allocation of participants into experimental groups is controlled but the process is not fully random nor fully concealed. |
| 3. Controlled Observations Studies<br>    3a. Cohort Studies<br>    3b. Case Control Studies | Studies in which the natural differences and variations between individuals or groups of participants are investigated, i.e. lung cancer rates amongst smokers. |
| 4. Observational Studies without Controls | As (3) above but without the controls. |
| 5. Expert Opinion (Clinical, Research, Consensus) | Papers that give expert opinion based on experience in either clinical practice, research or through consensus of a number of experts. |

## Growth in Nursing Literature?

Expansion of nursing journals.
Evidence-based practice.
Nursing research.

## Accessing the Literature: Databases

There is little point to having available the wealth of information that now exists regarding nursing if we are not able to access it in order to read it. There are a number of ways in which we can access the literature in a focused way.

## Learning Aid

Do I need help with my computer skills?

If you feel that your computer skills are inadequate then ask yourself where you can get help.

The librarian? Are there courses in the library to help you? Will you receive training in library skills as part of your course? Do you know someone who may be able to help you?

## Databases

As we have noted above there is now a voluminous amount of literature relating to all areas of healthcare practice and fortunately much of this is now stored on database retrieval systems. Prior to this, manual approaches to accessing the literature were the norm and journals and cataloguing systems were hand-searched for relevant articles. This meant scanning the journals for appropriate articles and then tracking down the references at the back to gather all the literature on a chosen topic. Although time consuming, this remains a good periodic practice, even after your electronic searches, in order to cross-reference and to ensure that the electronic databases have not missed a particular paper. This is particularly important with literature prior to the 1980s, when most databases were set up.

## Learning Aid

If you are unsure about how to access a database, do not ignore the problem but see above, 'Learning Aid'.

Don't put off using the computer in the library.

Don't think that you can complete your assignment by avoiding the literature searches. Your project will be impoverished — and so will your marks.

The databases vary in focus, but they basically undertake to scan thousands of journals and index the articles for bibliographic information and abstract details. Two examples are given below.

- MEDLINE (PUBMED). This database is produced by the US National Library of Medicine and is widely regarded as the main source for coverage of biomedical literature. It covers information from *Index Medicus*, *Index to Dental Literature* and *International Nursing*. It also covers information from areas of allied health, biological and physical sciences, humanities in relation to healthcare, and many areas related to medicine. It currently has 9.5 million records from more than 3,900 journals, as well as other source material.

- CINAHL (Cumulative Index to Nursing and Allied Health). This database provides authoritative coverage of the literature related to nursing and allied health. It claims to cover virtually all English-language nursing publications and in total indexes more than 500 journals and accesses books, conferences, dissertations and standards of practice.

## Learning Aid

How many other databases do I know of?
Where can I find information on them?
Do I have a friend who can attempt a database search with me?

As we say above, there are now many such databases, each covering a specific focus; for example, Box 4:3 gives an example of such healthcare-related databases – but reader beware, there are many more.

## Box 4:3    Examples of Electronic Databases

| Databases | Focus |
| --- | --- |
| EBM Reviews | Evidence-based medicine |
| Cochrane Database of Systematic Reviews | Restricted to systematic reviews |
| Database of Abstracts of Reviews | Focuses on effectiveness of interventions |
| Medline (PUBMED) | Main general healthcare database |
| Ovid Health STAR | Many areas covered including technology |
| CancerLit | Focuses on cancer therapy |
| AMED | Allied and complementary medicine |
| CINAHL | Nursing and allied professions |
| EMBASE | Biomedical and pharmaceutical |
| PsycINFO | Psychology, psychiatry, mental health |
| Cochrane Controlled Trials | Focuses on controlled trials |

Most colleges and university libraries have the facility to access these databases and an early trip to your friendly librarian is highly recommended. Information on managing the technology of these databases was outlined in Chapter 3.

## Accessing Databases?

Medline (PUBMED).

CINAHL.

Many others available.

## Learning Aid

You have spent a considerable amount of time gathering your references, so make sure that you secure them in a file. They are easily lost.

# Accessing the Literature: Focusing

## Overlap and Search Strategies

We can see from the foregoing that there must be considerable overlap of these databases, and indeed there is. This is particularly so if the topic being searched is a general one or the terms being used are not specific enough. However, if the topic under scrutiny is very specific (for example, complementary medicine or forensic mental health) then overlap is likely to be less of a problem. The secret of effective searching of electronic databases is the use of appropriate words to undertake the search and then the cross-referencing of searches to produce narrower fields. However, before we move on to explore search strategies it is worth mentioning that overlap not only occurs within healthcare databases but can also occur across other discipline databases. For example, articles in the journal *Sociology of Health* can be cross-referenced in healthcare databases as well as sociological ones. Therefore, beware of overlap, but also be aware that other databases may need to be searched.

Searching the electronic databases can be as simple or as complex as one wishes, and many of them are now in a standardised, or at least similar, format. Complex search strategies are a skill that you may need to develop over time but here we will focus on the basics of 'getting started'. Each library will have its own system of logging in to the computer and the password system to be employed. Therefore, you need to check with the librarians if you are unfamiliar with their system. Once logged on and a database has been chosen there is usually a box in which you type a word that you wish the computer to search for. If you choose a general word such as 'Nursing', then literally thousands of hits (records) will be located. Therefore, the computer will usually offer you a choice of more specific categories such as 'Nursing practice', 'Nursing education', 'Nursing research', and so on. Once you have decided which ones you wish to choose (you may choose as many as you wish) there will usually be another choice of whether to opt for 'explode' or 'focus'. This refers to whether the choice that you have made (e.g. Nursing practice) is a term that is merely mentioned in the paper (explode) or the term is the main focus of the paper (focus). Thus, we can see that we are beginning to narrow the search down a little.

## Learning Aid

There is overlap across databases.
Start with simple search strategies.
Mesh terms together.

Let's say that we wish to search for literature on the nursing practice of someone with Down syndrome. Now, if we take a more specific term, such as 'Down syndrome' and make this our second search term we will also get a considerable number of hits. Although we could focus our request more specifically to Trisomy, Translocation and Mosaic Down syndrome, we can leave it in its more general form for the moment. Thus we have two searches: (1) nursing practice and (2) Down syndrome. Our third, and more focused, search can now be made. This usually means typing into the search box '1 and 2', which is called 'meshing the terms'. The computer will now search for articles with both nursing practice and Down syndrome in the articles. There are other choices that can be made, such as whether to search for only those articles with an abstract and those that are research-based. This search will then give you references that are nursing practice and Down syndrome and are research-based.

## Learning Aid

A good abstract will provide a summary of a research paper, including aims, method, results and conclusion. You may be able to use this abstract instead of having to acquire the main paper. Using abstracts alone is dependent upon how well the summary has been produced by those creating the database. The abstract may not include important information that is in the paper, but which you will miss if you do not acquire the paper itself.

Finally, when searching for references, some related words begin with the same letters but the end letters differ, and the related terms may be lost if one of the full terms is used. For example, therapy, therapist and therapeutic all share the same letters up to 'therap', and if therapy is used as the search term, then therapist and therapeutic will be missed. Therefore, to include them all you need to type in 'therap*' (note the asterisk after all the shared letters) in some databases. This will then include therapy, therapist and therapeutic. An example of a simple search strategy can be seen in Box 4:4.

## Box 4:4    Simple Search Strategy

1.  Nursing practice
2.  Down syndrome
3.  1 and 2
4.  Nursing care
5.  2 and 4
6.  Challenging behaviour
7.  2 and 6
8.  1 and 2 and 6
9.  Therap*
10. 2 and 6 and 9

You may now carry on using narrower and narrower terms, and cross-reference them against each other until you have your desired focus and number of relevant articles. You can also see a display of short references only, which will include the title, author, source, volume, number and pages, or you can ask the computer to display other fields as well, such as abstract, reference list, etc.

## Need a Search Strategy?

Consider overlap of sources.
Try simple searches and complex ones.
Consider use of search terms.
Explode and focus.
Consider use of asterisk.

## Literature Reviews and Seminal Papers

In seeking to focus your literature review take care not to miss important papers. A useful tip is to search your topic area with the words 'review' and 'update', which will capture any references that have reviewed your field. It may be the case that some authors have published a paper titled 'A Review of the Nursing Care of Diabetic Patients', for example, or 'Nursing Care of Down Syndrome: A Literature Review'. If this is the case in the area of your search then it is vital that you acquire this article, for three main reasons. First, this author has done what you are attempting to do (i.e. a review of the literature) and you will be able to read much of the groundwork that you are covering. Therefore, what you will need to do, depending on how good their review is, is to update the review and probably expand it from the year of publication. Second, their reference list should be a comprehensive coverage of the literature and may contain some references that you have missed. Third, they will have given their review a structure of sub-headings, which you may find useful for your project or provide stimulation for your own structure. Therefore, the latest and best 'literature review/update' of your topic is a must to acquire.

## Need a Review Paper?

They have done what you are doing.
They will have produced a reference list.
They will have provided a structure.

Finally, when you are reading papers on your topic look out for any comment that suggests that a particular reference is a 'seminal paper'. Seminal papers are important to you and must be acquired. For a paper to be considered seminal it must have provided new and vital information, or an alternative interpretation, in your field and must be studied carefully and used in your project. When reading an article that is considered seminal try to pinpoint where it is saying something new and look for both the line of argument and the impact that it has had, or may have. You can then discuss these in your own work. We have focused on journal articles here as they are more commonly used, but searching for books and chapters in books can also be undertaken in the appropriate databases.

## Reviewing the Literature?

Acquire important papers.
Look for review papers.
Acquire seminal papers.
Look for a structure.

# Reading and Critiquing the Literature

Once you have chosen the references that you require from the searches that have been made, you need to acquire them, read them and critique them. In order to acquire the actual articles or books, first check whether your own library takes the journal or has the book in its stock. This information, again, may be held on a database, but if it is not, then ask the librarian. If the articles or books are in stock in the library then it is a simple matter of tracking them down via the referencing system. If they are not available in your own library, you can order them through your librarian, and this will usually require the filling out of a short form and in some cases the payment of a small charge. The journal articles may need to be photocopied. As the number of articles that you acquire grows they will need to be stored appropriately. Having gone to all that trouble of getting the articles, it is incredibly annoying to lose them and have to go and retrieve them once more, especially if you have to pay for them. Any system of management is appropriate if it works; therefore choose the one that serves you best. However, one system will be suggested here.

## Learning Aid

Ordering specific articles or books from a central source, such as the British Library, may take several weeks. Therefore, undertake your literature review and make your orders as soon as possible. Time is always short.

Write the main author's name and year of publication in the top right-hand corner of the front sheet of the paper as it would be filed in a lever-arch or box-type file. This allows for a quick leafing through when searching for a particular paper. Keep them in alphabetical order (by name of first author) both for easy referral and to marry up to the full reference list that you are compiling on index cards or on computer. Do not forget to copy the reference of the article onto your index card system (see below) or place them onto your computer database as you acquire the articles/books (if you have not already done so). If large volumes of articles are being amassed you may need to construct a sub-file system of lever-arch or box files. For example, diabetes references may need the sub-files of Growth Onset, Maturity Onset and Secondary/Non-hereditary files.

## Learning Aid

Effective management of the literature in a systematic and organised way will save time.

## Acquiring the Literature?

In the library stock?
If not, can you order them from the library?
Make photocopies.
Write the author's name on the front page at the top for ease of referencing.
Keep them in a file.

## Reading

Now you are ready to read, and we should note that there are different 'levels' or ways of reading a piece of work. First, there is 'scanning', in which you may be flipping through the paper looking for its structure of headings and sub-headings, reading a few sentences to get a 'feel' for the grammar, spelling and syntax, and getting an idea of its length and quality of referencing. 'Scanning' is a useful process to give you an indication of the overall structure and thrust of the article in relation to the sub-headings. Second, there is reading for meaning, which refers to studying the content of the article carefully to establish what the main arguments are – in short, what the authors mean to say, by your interpretation. Third, there is reading for sense, that is, identifying whether the article makes sense in relation to their analysis of issues, their line of argumentation, their interpretation of information and the conclusions that they draw. Finally, there is reading for research. Although all types of reading contribute towards an overall critique of the literature, it is this last type of reading that requires the greatest skill (more on this below). Before you begin to read there are a couple of items that you may find helpful – highlighter pens, a pencil and an eraser, but remember only to use them on your *own* copy.

## Learning Aid

Scanning literature and looking for relevant references to support your work
is a skill. The more you do it, the better you become at it. But it comes with
a warning. If you rely on scanning only, then you may miss important information.

As you begin to read you can use the coloured highlighter pens for a coding system to link into different things. For example, you may use one colour to highlight research matters such as numbers, percentages, statistics, methods, sample, analysis, and so on. Another colour can be used to signal an important or interesting comment that you may use as a quote, and another colour to mark any references that you may need to acquire to add to your list. The pencil can be used to write any notes in the margin that you may need to follow-up or question in your critique. Highlighting and making notes will save you time later when you are writing up your project. You will develop your own system and style as you progress and you will become more proficient the more you read. Just as in seeing a film for the second time one may notice something that was missed in the first viewing, so it can be in the second reading of an article. Therefore, you need to read it at least twice, but preferably with a little passage of time between readings.

## Learning Aid

Highlight important points.
Write down notes.
Summarise main points of the paper.
Index cards.
What is the coding system that you are using?
Can you change it as you go along?
How will it influence the structure of your assignment?

After the first reading you can then go through your highlighted material and notes and write them on either your reference index card or a separate sheet of paper which can be attached to the article in its file or kept in a separate file. This will make the writing up of your project a simple matter of taking out the specific information that you require and you will not need to plough through the entire article each time (see Box 4:5).

## Box 4:5    Example of Index Card of Fictitious Study

Smith, J. (1999) An examination of breast cancer in a fictitious female population. *Journal of Pretence Nursing*, 34(6): 45–54.

    Good study but has limitations. Undertaken in Greenland. Postal survey
    Total population 300 female subjects
    Return rate 50% ($n = 150$)
    10% ($n = 15$) with breast cancer
    8 improved with example drug
    Limitations to study, PTO

## Critiquing

We will now look at critiquing the literature in relation to research papers, which requires specific skills as mentioned above. The critique of a research paper follows the traditional structure of the research process itself and the more knowledgeable you are of this the more able you will be in critiquing a research study. Box 4:6 outlines the research process and suggests some questions that might be posed.

### Box 4:6   Critiquing a Research Paper

| Process | Questions |
|---|---|
| Title | Does it make sense? Does it relate to the content of the paper? Is it concise? Has it a research focus? |
| Author | Do they have the necessary qualifications? Is it their area of professional expertise? |
| Abstract | Is it succinct? Is it structured appropriately according to type of paper, e.g. research or feature article, etc.? Does it summarise the study? |
| Introduction | Is it broad enough to introduce the topic? Are the problems clearly established? Does it end in the specific focus of the paper? |
| Background | Does it provide a context? Would the non-specialist have a better focus after reading? |
| Literature Review | Is the literature well covered? Are many sources used? Are central or seminal works noted? Is it logically structured? Is it up to date? Is there a theoretical or conceptual framework? Is it balanced or prejudiced? Is the need for their current paper clearly established? Does it lead logically to the Aims, etc.? |
| AOHQ (Aims/Objectives/ Hypotheses/Questions) | Are they clearly stated? Check if more than one relationship is made in each hypothesis (there should be only one). Can the hypothesis be realistically tested? |
| Method | Is the method stated? Is it appropriate to meet the AOHQ? Is there a discussion of strengths and weaknesses? |
| Population | Is the population specified? |

*(Continued)*

| | |
|---|---|
| Sample | Is the sampling unit stated? Is the sampling frame appropriate? Are the figures appropriate? Are the figures explained? Is the sampling frame generalisable to the population? |
| Data Collection | Is the type of data to be collected reported? |
| Data Management | Is this explained in terms of what, where, when and how? |
| Data Analysis | Is this explained clearly? Does it fit with the type of data collected? Does this achieve the requirements of the Aims/Hypotheses, etc.? |
| Ethics | Are research committees mentioned, e.g. Local Research Ethics Committee/Multi-site Research Ethics Committee? Is confidentiality observed? Is anonymity explained? Is the Data Protection Act mentioned? Is the data secured? |
| Results | Are they stated clearly? Do they link into the data analysis? Are they appropriately reported? |
| Discussion | Is this balanced? Does it emanate from the analysis and results? Are the Aims/Hypotheses, etc., adequately dealt with? Does it deal with previous research papers adequately? |
| Conclusions/ Recommendations | Are these drawn logically from the study? Are they realistic? |
| Limitations of Study | Are these mentioned? To what extent do they limit the study? Can they be overcome in future research? |
| References | Are they there? Are they accurately completed? |
| Appendices | Are they included? Are they appropriate? |

Obviously not all these questions will relate to every study, but serve as a guide in working through research papers. Attempt to follow the arguments in the papers and ascertain what the main points are that are being made. Summarise the study for yourself.

## Critiquing the Literature?

Read the paper several times.

Follow the research process.

Be sceptical.

Know the difference between critique and criticism.

# How to Write a Literature Review

Once you have read all the literature, made notes from reading and re-reading and highlighting the relevant information, you are now in a position to write your literature review. It may be that you are going to use a structure from one of your journal articles or book chapters, or it may be that you are going to develop your own structure. If the latter is the case and you are having difficulty creating one, there are a few tips that may help you.

## Learning Aid

Types of research design (see Box 4.2).
Types of the condition (e.g. Trisomy, Translocation and Mosaic Down syndrome)
Types of care (e.g. nursing, medical, physiotherapy, occupational therapy, alternative)
Course of the condition (e.g. aetiology, signs and symptoms, interventions, prognosis)

Once you have your structure it is now just a matter of inserting your references within the structure as they fit. For example, suppose your structure included a sub-heading of 'treatment outcome' and you have a number of articles in which this is reported, these can now be incorporated into your review.

## Box 4:7   Literature Review Construction

Treatment Outcome (sub-heading of structure)
There are numerous studies in which treatment outcomes have been reported, some positively and some negatively. For example, Green (2004) reported that 74 percent of patients positively responded to the treatment. This was supported by Brown (2005) who recorded 76 percent and Smith (2005) with an even higher figure of 78 percent. Others have reported positive results but not this high level (Mason, 2006; Whitehead, 2006). However, negative results have also been noted by ... and so on.

Finally, time to write a literature review will be mentioned. Undertaking literature reviews is a time-consuming activity, from start to finish, particularly in relation to searching, acquiring and reading the material. However, writing up the review is also time-consuming and you need to be able to put time aside to undertake the writing (see Chapter 2). Do not be put off starting, and once underway you will find it a relatively simple task to keep inserting your articles as they are assessed – as long as you read, re-read and take notes.

# Conclusions

With the increasing volume of literature that is being produced, and which is set to continue, the skill of being able to manage this material has grown, and is continuing to grow, in importance. Although there is a tremendous amount of documentation to be covered it is important not to be daunted by this. We have seen that there are skills and techniques now available which assist us in managing the literature. As is the case with most things in life, the more you do something the more skilled you become in doing it, and it is the same with accessing, managing, reading and critiquing the wide and varied publications on any given topic in today's modern healthcare setting.

## SUMMARY POINTS OF CHAPTER 4

- It is important to understand the relevance of supporting literature.
- The huge growth in literature means that there is a wide variety of sources from which to access it.
- Reviewing the literature is important and may include scanning and reading for meaning, sense and research.
- Literature reviews are used in many areas of studentship, including essays, assignments, projects and research.

# Test Your Study Skills ...

1. What are the key issues to consider when using literature to support your abstract? (see page 68)

2. What is meant by the theoretical framework for managing the literature? (see page 64)

3. What are (a) primary sources, and (b) secondary sources, of literature? (see page 61)

4. Name two databases that specifically deal with nursing literature? (see page 66)

5. What is the difference between a primary source of literature and a secondary source of literature (see page 61)

6. How would you catalogue your given subject? (see page 69)

## Practical Session ...

Choose a subject that you are interested in and ...

1. Access the databases using a simple search strategy (see page 69).

2. Categorise the literature as explained (see page 63).

3. Write a brief summary of your literature search using sub-headings to provide a structure (see pages 70, 72 and 76).

# 5 Assignment Writing

## Introduction

Writing essays and assignments will be vitally important in most courses of study and nursing is no exception. Furthermore, nurses are increasingly being called upon to write projects of one description or another in many areas of nursing. This often causes tension, particularly for those who are not used to writing, or may not have written anything for a long time. We will discuss students' vulnerability in this chapter and examine a number of rules that should be followed before beginning. We will also highlight how avoidance strategies operate to prevent us from writing and discuss ways in which these can be used positively. Planning assignments should be undertaken carefully and we outline how to structure various projects, essays and reports. Writers' block and the fear of the blank page often cause students difficulty and we will discuss how to overcome these problems. Finally, we will emphasise the importance of recension, which refers to the reading and re-reading of your own work for checking and editing.

## Types of Theoretical Assessments

Students entering higher education today will be faced with a range of theoretical assessments. These assessments are designed to test various aspects of students' knowledge and their ability to demonstrate their critical thinking skills. There are a number of reasons for the increase in different types of theoretical assessments. First, there is a recognition that the traditional essays and exams can only test specific ways of learning. For example, exams, as every student knows, rely upon the recall of a reservoir of knowledge that students have acquired in their revision and then are able to demonstrate that knowledge on the appropriate day. Second, lecturers recognize that students are not a homogeneous group and while some are good at exams others shine in essays and other forms of assessments. Therefore, a variety of theoretical assessments will capture the vast array of strengths that students have and allow for the expression of knowledge in different ways. Third, lecturers are concerned that they use the most appropriate type of assessment to 'test' the subject under assessment. For example, multiple-choice questions can be employed to assess students' knowledge of the use of different treatments for particular conditions. However, multiple-choice questions would not be able to test the analytical depth required to assess the nature of caring.

## The Importance of Essays and Assignments

Although you may well not agree with us at this moment in time, writing your essay or assignment is an exciting point in the process of studying. It is exciting and important, because this is the point at which you can display all the hard work that you have been doing over the previous weeks, months or even years. You have, or should have, organised your study, learnt how to use modern-day technology, amassed your reading material, spent long hours reading and synthesising the literature, and acquired a considerable amount of knowledge. It may have been difficult learning so much as you have gone along, juggling so many things around to placate family and friends. You have probably moaned to others about your workload and lack of time to fit everything in, and you have probably been moaned at for not being readily available and for spending all your time studying! A lot of studying time is invisible to others, especially tutors and lecturers, as they do not 'see' you in the long lonely hours of your endeavour. But now it is your turn to show them the evidence of your efforts, it is your turn to display to them the knowledge that you have gained, and it is your turn to be visible – very visible! This, naturally, causes some trepidation, as you must now reveal what you know.

## Writing?

Show them what you can do.
Visibility is vulnerability.

In producing a written piece of work it may be that you feel an element of vulnerability. Perhaps you feel that your knowledge base is insufficient to do justice to the assignment or perhaps you feel that you have sufficient knowledge but that you cannot express it articulately. Furthermore, you may believe that the written work you produce will be laughed at or ridiculed, because you think that others will feel that it is badly written and look childish. These are natural feelings that we all feel and it is only through practice that we gain confidence to overcome them and write our projects up. Box 5:1 indicates a number of the more common things that we have heard students say; however, there are many more.

## Box 5:1    Some Excuses for Not Writing

- I'm still reading around the subject.
- I don't know enough.
- I can't express what I know.
- They will think I'm stupid.
- I can't write.
- They will see that I can't write.
- My spelling is awful.
- I've nothing to say.
- I don't know how to write.
- My grammar and punctuation are poor.
- I can't get started.
- I don't want to write, I just want to nurse.
- And so on ...

In a practical profession such as nursing you may question why it is that you are asked to write. Well, one obvious answer is that you need to write in order to reveal your knowledge so that you can pass your exams. Another reason is that you will be called upon to communicate patient care and patient progress via the written record constantly throughout your career. You may join a branch of nursing that requires you to produce reports for case conferences or even courts (for example, health visitors).

However, there is another reason for honing your writing skills, and that is a question of professionalism. You may go on to write articles for publication or even a book such as this one. You may do research and need to construct a research report for dissemination or join a committee and be required to contribute towards an official report. Or, you may decide that you want to go on to further study and need to produce more essays. In any event, do not be under any illusion that modern-day nursing is merely a practical endeavour alone. It is not, and is unlikely to be so in a society that requires professionals to be legally accountable.

## Why is Writing Important?

Reveals your knowledge.

Communication.

Produce reports.

Professionalism.

Publications.

## Rules of the Road

Writing is a skill similar to driving a car. Yes, there are gifted writers, just as there are gifted drivers, but the vast majority of us are ordinary motorists who have learnt the basics of driving, follow the rules of the road (well, nearly always), successfully navigate our journey and arrive at our destination. Writing is a similar process. However, remember when you first got into a car to learn how to drive and how complicated everything felt. How on earth would you ever be able to co-ordinate the mirrors, the steering, the clutch, the gears, the accelerator and, most importantly, the brakes? Now, you probably jump into the car and get from A to B, and probably do not remember managing all the components of driving. Writing too has several components to it, which, when learnt individually and then put together into one operation, produce a quality end product. This chapter sets out these components, but before we venture out, there are certain rules of the 'highway code' that we need to be aware of (see Box 5:2).

## Remember?

Writing is like driving a car.

It has several components to it.

Learnt and practised equals pleasant journey.

## Box 5:2   Rules of the Road

- Understand the assignment.
- Understand what is being asked for.
- Establish the deadline.
- Find out where the information is.
- Produce a logical argument.

The first rule is to ensure that you understand the assignment brief. There are many ways of writing and there are many different writing styles. We will outline four basic types that you are likely to encounter during the course of your study. The first style is termed *descriptive*, but this is a general term indicating numerous approaches within it. For example, you may be called upon to *describe* a series of events or *describe* the main features of a particular report. Descriptive writing is a portrayal of the main features of whatever you are writing about. The second style of writing is termed *analytical*, which has two main aspects to it: (a) argumentative and (b) evaluative. *Analytical argumentative* writing involves stating a point, providing some evidence, contrasting this with other evidence and interpretations, and drawing logical conclusions from this. In *analytical evaluative* writing, which is not too dissimilar, you need to compare and contrast issues, points of view, validity of evidence, styles, approaches or methods. You also need to establish the similarities of points of significance and any implications drawn from them. Finally, you will need to make judgements or draw conclusions and in doing so you will need to establish the criteria that you have adopted for making them. The final style of writing is referred to as *anecdotal*, which draws on the author's personal experience or their interpretation of someone else's personal experience.

## Writing Styles?

Descriptive.
Analytical argumentative.
Analytical evaluative.
Anecdotal.

## Learning Aid

Using personal experience without supportive evidence is often criticised by markers. Avoid the personal pronoun 'I' except in reflective writing.

Care has to be taken with the reflective style of writing as it can be criticised for lack of academic style. If using this style of writing avoid the personal pronoun 'I' and use 'this author' or 'this writer' instead. Also, try to incorporate research evidence in support of your personal statements.

The second rule is to make sure that you understand what is being asked for. Often students produce wonderful essays about a particular topic, only to discover that they were not asked to write about that and are marked down accordingly. Read and re-read the question being asked, or assignment topic, several times and write it out in your own words to see if you have the same emphasis as in the question. The third rule is to establish the deadline. Make sure that you understand when the assignment is to be submitted and how much time you have to complete it. This will determine your plan of attack (see Chapter 1). The fourth rule is to establish where the information is that you require and how you can access it.

## Learning Aid

Do not fall into the trap of believing that you have plenty of time — you don't! Start immediately, find out where the information is and acquire it. Make notes as you are reading.

The final rule to be mentioned here is to produce a logical argument or line of reasoning. This entails producing evidence for a particular argument and establishing reasonable cause and effect.

There are, of course, many more rules to writing and the five mentioned here are merely the main ones to get you started, and as you work through this chapter you will note many other rules to guide you.

## Avoidance Strategies

Much of the process of writing concerns acquiring the literature, getting information, visiting the library, reading the material, sorting, organising and planning. However, there comes a point when you know full well that it is time to sit down and begin writing. You are aware that you should actually be putting pen to paper as the deadline is approaching. Yet most people avoid doing so until the very last minute. At one level avoiding writing is unconscious and the person does not explicitly know that they are avoiding it, as they employ a series of rationalisations as a form of denial. The human mind has what are known as defence mechanisms, which are psychological strategies to protect a person's ego or self-esteem. Some are conscious and some are unconscious; that is, in some we are aware that we are employing them and in others we are not. In avoiding the moment that we actually sit down and write we are defending our mind against the uncomfortable real-isation that we lack confidence in writing. The lack of confidence produces a tension in us and we avoid it through a process of rationalising doing anything but writing. There are as many avoidance strategies as there are human excuses, and they are only restricted by the human imagination. They tend to fall into two main types with the first having some form of time dimension and the second being a question of prioritisation.

The time-avoidance strategies involve a form of watershed or natural break in the calendar. For example, when coming up to Christmas we may say to ourselves 'I will start straight away in the new year', or when the children are on school holidays we may think 'I will start the moment that they go back to school'. Box 5:3 outlines a few other common time-avoidance strategies.

## Avoidance Strategies?

Can be conscious or unconscious processes.
May employ time or priorities.

## Box 5:3    Time-Avoidance Strategies

- It's too late now. I'll start first thing in the morning.
- The sun's shining at the moment. I'll do it when it's raining.
- It's Friday afternoon. I'll start first thing on Monday morning.
- It's Saturday. I'll start Sunday.
- It's nearly the end of the month. I'll start on the first of next month.
- My partner/children is/are going away next week. I'll do it then.
- And so on ...

The second set of avoidance strategies employs a series of prioritisations and are very interesting to analyse as they can be quite serious activities or they can be extremely trivial. We employ them to avoid writing by prioritising other activities above sitting down and putting pen to paper. They usually occur when we have made the time to write but allow another activity to be done before we begin to write. They are usually rationalised with the mental thoughts, or actual words: 'I'll just do ... (whatever) ... before starting to write.' They may include 'I'll just do the shopping and then I'll start' or 'I'll just feed the dog and then I'll begin.' Box 5:4 highlights a few of the more common priority-avoidance strategies.

## Box 5:4    Priority-Avoidance Strategies

I'll just ...
- make a phone call,
- mow the lawn,
- tidy the shed,

*(Continued)*

*(Continued)*

- tidy the drawer,
- sharpen the pencils,
- rearrange the books,
- change the bed,
- do the washing,
- do the ironing,
- make a cup of tea,

... and then I'll start.

## Learning Aid

What are your main avoidance strategies? Write them down on a piece of paper.

Identifying what your avoidance strategies are is important, as only through revealing them, and bringing them into full consciousness, will you be able to adequately address them. So, know your avoidance strategies and when you find yourself engaging in one of them highlight it by telling yourself (preferably out loud) that 'this is an avoidance strategy'. This emphasises the fact, gives you a guilty conscience and allows you to correct it. When you have identified your avoidance strategies you can then turn them into a type of 'reward' for writing. We suggest that if you are about to start writing and find yourself saying 'I'll just ... before starting' you should say to yourself 'I will write ... (one sentence, one paragraph or one page) ... and then I will ... (make a cup of tea, tidy the drawer, go to the pub).' By changing the avoidance strategy into a type of reward you force yourself to begin writing before your other activity and in effect re-prioritise and avoid avoiding.

There are, of course, other factors that contribute towards not writing and we will address the two most common problems: (a) the mental block and (b) the blank page. All writers suffer from mental block at some stage or another, and in academic writing this is usually accompanied by the terrifying thought 'I've nothing to say.' Of course you have – it just needs to be extracted, and there are mechanisms available to assist you in this. The major mechanism to overcome blocking is to plan the assignment in detail, and this is covered in the next section. However, we can outline a few other ways to overcome this problem here. The first is to talk it through, out loud, either to yourself or to someone else. Imagine explaining it to a young child in order to simplify it. Second, break up the project into smaller manageable chunks (see 'Planning' below) and start anywhere in the project where you feel comfortable. Remember that only you will see the early drafts of your work so do not be afraid of making mistakes at this stage. Third, brainstorm your ideas on a flip chart, whiteboard or piece of paper. Doodle and draw if it helps and scribble down anything and everything that might be related. Use diagrams, questions, lists, cartoons, networks or any illustrations you can think of to map out your ideas. Finally, break the tension and relax by getting up and walking around, make that cup of tea, stretch and keep talking to yourself.

## The Mental Block?

Can be overcome by planning, talking, breaking into smaller parts, brainstorming and relaxing.
Scribble, doodle or draw on the blank page.

Finally, we will address the blank page. Recently we had cause to observe an artist begin a painting. He sat down at his easel and placed a white canvas upon it. He took up his palette and brushes, and looked at the canvas. He said out loud 'I hate the whiteness of the blank canvas, so let's get rid of it.' He took up his largest brush and aggressively squiggled the colour light blue all over the canvas and then said 'now we can start'. In writing circles, dealing with the blank page is similar. If a blank page bothers you, try writing in pencil so that you can rub it out. Scribble down ideas on it, or put a doodle somewhere on it and write around it. Write on loose paper rather than in a book so that you can try various approaches, and use or change the words when you type it up. If a blank page is problematic then make it not blank as quickly as possible by putting anything on it as did our artist above who went on to cover the blue with a beautiful painting. The lesson is that what you first put down is not the finished product.

# Planning

No matter what you are writing, planning is the single most important aspect and its emphasis cannot be stressed enough. Whether you are writing an advertisement, a letter, an essay, a thesis or a book, the planning of it is of paramount importance. It is important for two fundamental reasons. The first is that you need to plan so that you incorporate all the components that you need to, and second, when you plan you are actually writing the project in your mind. As we write this book we have before us a detailed plan on one side of A3 paper with all the chapters and their sub-headings written down, and within the sub-headings we have a series of bullet points to indicate what material we wish to cover. Although the plan for a book of 80,000 words is naturally bigger than a plan for an assignment of 2,500 words, they are the same in structure. Now let us look at how we plan a particular project in a little more detail.

The first planning strategy is to establish the length of your work and the number of words you write on a sheet of paper. Although some people can sit at a computer and write by typing straight onto the screen, most prefer to sit at a desk and write on paper first. So, assuming that you are going to write your assignment in pencil or pen first, and then type it later, you need to know how many words you write, on average, on each page. This will depend on how many lines there are on the page and how small your writing is. Some people write on every second line and leave the blank lines for corrections or additions. It doesn't really matter as long as you find a system that you are comfortable with and stick to it. Once you know how many words you write on a page then you can work out how many pages you will need to complete your project. For example, if you write approximately 300 words per page, and your essay needs to be 1,200 words in length, then you know that you will need four pages of written work. You are normally allowed plus or minus 10 per cent of the wordage so the range of your project will be between 1,080 and 1,320 words. When you come to type up your essay remember that the typed words per A4 page, with font 12-point Times Roman, single line spacing, is approximately 500 words.

The second strategy is to establish your deadline and to work out how many words you need to write per day, ensuring that you allow for typing, reading over your project, editing, re-reading and preparing for presentation. However, if you focus on your actual writing time you need to work out how many words need to be written per day. Don't forget to give yourself some leeway and some time off. The most important thing is to be realistic and make it achievable. Box 5:5 shows a basic working out for a 2,500-word essay, which is to be presented in one month, assuming that all the literature has been read.

## Planning Assignment

Number of words on page.
Number of pages in project.

## Planning Towards Deadline?

Plan start to finish.
Number of words per day.
Give yourself some leeway.

The third aspect to your plan is to establish a series of headings and sub-headings, and make sure that you keep a consistent framework in using upper case (capital letters) and lower case (small letters), bold, underline, italics, bullet points and numbering. Box 5:6 shows a common framework for a heading and sub-heading structure.

The next step in your plan is to identify a structure. Take a moment and look at the content pages of this book. When we sat down to think about writing this book we scribbled down the chapter headings, with each chapter on a separate piece of paper, and then put a series of sub-headings in each chapter to give it an overall structure. Then we put some bullet points in each sub-section to show what the content might look like. Over the months we adjusted and re-adjusted the structure, adding and subtracting, until finally we had the structure that you see before you. All projects, no matter how big or how small, need to have a structure of one sort or another.

## Box 5:5  Working out Wordage for an Essay

2 weeks' writing time = 14 days.
2 weekends off = 10 writing evenings.
2,500-word essay/10 evenings = 250 words per evening.
@ 250 written words per page = one written page per evening.
10 written pages required to complete the project.

**Recension**
First re-read and edit = 3 days.
Second re-read and edit = 1 day.
Prepare for presentation = 1 day.

## Learning Aid

Although you have some leeway as to how you structure your project there are some basic requirements that are more than likely to be needed. For example, all projects require an introduction at the beginning and most need a conclusion at the end.

## Box 5:6    Headings and Sub-headings with Emphasis

**TITLE** (Upper case and bold)
**Introduction** (Upper/lower case and bold)
**Literature Review** (Upper/lower case and bold)
  Published Material (Underline)
   *Journals* (Italics)
   *Books* (Italics)
   *Other Material* (Italics)
  Official Reports (Underline)
   *Pre-1970* (Italics)
   *1971–2000* (Italics)
   *Post-2000* (Italics)
  Anecdotal Evidence (Underline)
   *Anonymous Accounts* (Italics)
   *Personal Experience* (Italics)
  Other Source Material (Underline)
   *MSc Theses* (Italics)
   *PhD Theses* (Italics)
**Conclusions** (Upper/lower case and bold)
**References** (Upper/lower case and bold)

Box 5:7 shows a structure for a short essay on violence in healthcare settings, of 4,000 words in length.

## Box 5:7    Structure and Wordage for an Essay

Title: Violence in Healthcare Settings
Introduction (200 words)
Background (300 words)
Literature Review (1,500 words)
  Historical Material (500)

*(Continued)*

Research Papers (500)
Official Reports (500)
Conclusions (250 words)
Recommendations (250 words)
References
   **Total Words = 4,000**

Note the loading of the number of words for each section, with the main body of the essay having the major number of words. Many courses in universities and colleges have a set requirement for the structuring of your project so you need to check with the course leaders or the course handbook before deciding on your structure. If you are producing a research paper then this tends to have a set series of sub-headings (see Box 5:8). The number of words is a rough guide only and will vary according to the journal that the paper is being sent to.

## Box 5:8    Basic Structure of a Research Paper

Title
Abstract (150)
Introduction (400)
Background/Context (400)
Literature Review (1,500)
Aims or Objectives or Research Questions or Hypotheses (150)
Method (300)
Results (500)
Discussion (2,000)
Conclusions and Recommendations (300)
References
   **Total Words = 5,700**

Depending upon what you are presenting and the size of the project, you may need to choose a structure that incorporates all the sub-headings of an official report. These can be seen in Box 5:9.

# Box 5:9   Components of a Report

**Title:** This should be as succinct as possible and relate to your project. It should be understandable by others. It should stand alone in the middle of the first page with your name and course underneath it. A contact address should be supplied if you are writing an article for publication.

**Contents Page:** A full list of the contents including acknowledgements, preface, references, list of tables and illustrations, appendices and index.

**Acknowledgements:** Mention all those who have assisted you in some way or another. Don't become too emotional. Acknowledgements can come at the end of a research paper if you are mentioning those who have awarded the research grant.

**Preface:** This is usual in a book and you should explain why the book is necessary and the reasons for its production.

**Foreword:** This is written by someone else rather than the author or contributor. They are usually recognised experts in the area that the book covers.

**Abstract:** A short paragraph that summarises your project or research. It should contain aims, method, main findings and conclusion.

**Introduction:** This should start with broad general statements and then finish more focused, and relate it to your current project.

**Background:** This should set your work in context and give reasons why the work is being done and its importance.

**Literature Review:** This should be comprehensive and cover all the relevant material you are aware of published and unpublished. It should be structured into a series of sub-headings that covers all the areas. Draw out all the relevant research and the main findings. Relate this to your work. It should finish by identifying any gaps in the knowledge base and should indicate why your study is necessary.

**Aims or Objectives or Research Questions or Hypotheses:** These should come out of the literature review and should be clearly stated.

**Method:** This should be clearly stated and be designed to address the aims, objectives, etc. It can have sub-headings to include the population, the data to be collected, the data management, the data analysis, and inclusion and exclusion criteria.

**Ethical Implications:** Briefly mention any ethical implications and how these are managed. You should mention confidentiality, anonymity, informed consent, research committees, the Data Protection Act, and how you will protect the data.

*(Continued)*

**Results:** This is usually a short section. These should be presented briefly and without discussing them. You can present them as they arose from your analysis or put them in order of importance.

**Discussion:** This is a longer section and should be organised to address your aims, objectives, etc. You should take your main findings and discuss them in relation to existing research or locate them in relation to a particular theory. You need to discuss whether they were expected, their relevance and importance, and their significance to practice.

**Limitations to the Study:** Briefly mention the limitations to your study and how these could be rectified in further research.

**Conclusions:** Summarise your main findings and make a statement regarding whether your aims, objectives, etc., have been met.

**Recommendations:** If relevant you need to make a series of recommendations for policy development or practice delivery. Make them short and succinct, and make them achievable.

**References:** A full list of all references that you have used should be provided in alphabetical order.

**Appendices:** These should be numbered according to how you have referred to them in the main text. They are usually copies of instruments that have been used, letters to participants, relevant materials and other data not presented in the main text.

You may not use all these components in a project but they are useful, as you can pick from them and make your own structure according to the type of project that you are undertaking. Finally, once you have chosen your structure you can begin to plan what the content is likely to be.

## Learning Aid

The more detailed your plan, the easier the writing-up will be.

Pick from the options of headings.

Set it out in a series of sub-headings.

Use bullet points for each paragraph.

# Writing

Once you have overcome the avoidance strategies and have organised a detailed plan you should now be ready to sit down and write your first words. Remember, you can start anywhere in the project and only you will see the first draft so do not be too worried about spelling and grammar at this stage. Take one of your bullet points from your plan and tackle the writing in short paragraphs. The first sentence in your paragraph should introduce the topic of your paragraph whilst the middle sentences should develop the theme. Make sure that the sentences are set out in a logical order and are linked to each other, and the final sentence should sum up the paragraph accordingly. Take your time to think what the point of the paragraph is that you are writing and then what each sentence should say. There should be a link between each sentence and the sentences should be concise. Write in the third person (except in reflective accounts) by using phrases such as 'it was found that …', rather than 'I found that …'.

Writing is similar to sculpting and the words are pieces of 'clay' to be manipulated. Therefore, once you have written a paragraph or section you need to type it into a word-processing package. Take this opportunity to make this your first editing process. As you type, read the sentence back to yourself. Continue this until you have a full paragraph or section typed in. Then print a copy out and read it from the page. Make a note of any changes you wish to make and read it as if you were a stranger reading it for the first time. Read it out loud and ask yourself whether it makes sense, whether it reads well, could be improved and makes the point that you wish to make. Remember it is 'clay' and can be changed, altered and restructured until the paragraph, section and project is crafted into the shape that you want. Continue this until your assignment is written in full.

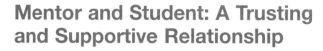

## Writing

Is like sculpting.
Words are like clay.

# Mentor and Student: A Trusting and Supportive Relationship

Students may have a number of mentors, who may include your Personal Academic Tutor (these roles may be separated into Academic Tutor and Personal Tutor), Module Leader, Programme Leader and Clinical Mentor. Whatever title they have, the role of the mentor is to support the student – that's you! As a student in higher education it is largely up to you to make appointments to see your mentor(s). In terms of writing your assignment we suggest you prepare to see your mentor in advance:

1. Check the tutorial time you are allocated (this should be in your programme/module handbook).
2. Make a note of your allocated mentor. Send them an email and introduce yourself.
3. Your mentor may have tutorial times where you can make an appointment – do this as soon as possible.
4. Take questions to the tutorial and make notes. Your mentor will probably give you notes at the end of the meeting.
5. If you cannot make the tutorial – notify your mentor and make another appointment – we advise you to take full advantage of tutorial support.

# The Process of Writing and Submitting Your Assignment

## Stage 1: The Assignment Details

- This usually takes place in the first week of your module. The assignment details are generally given to the students by your module leader, who will be happy to assist you with any questions that you may have.
- Read the assignment details carefully and note down the following:

    a)    The question or area to be covered.
    b)    The word length.
    c)    Any additional information.

- Note down the submission date and the re-submission date (hopefully you won't need this!)
- Remember to use your tutorial time and make your appointment to see your tutor early.

## Stage 2: The Preparation Phase

- Start your preparation to-day! It is tempting when you receive your submission date of 22nd January on 4th October to be lulled into a false sense of security. It may seem like a long time away, but Christmas and New Year will come all too soon and you'll be thinking of excuses for requesting an extension to the submission date!
- Students often complain and argue that they cannot start their assignment until they've been taught something. We disagree! You can begin jotting down ideas, visiting the library and reading around the subject area.
- Commence your literature search and begin to manage your literature (see Chapter 4).
- If you think that you may need additional support with study skills, we urge you to make an appointment with your module leader or personal academic tutor as soon as possible, and we can assure you that other students will be in a similar position. Sometimes the support that you require may be quite modest, or you may be a student who feels that something quite significant needs attention.

- Most students have to plan for at least one or two assignments to be submitted at the same time, so planning ahead is very important.
- If you think you are going to run into problems with your assignment schedule, contact your module leader or personal academic tutor as soon as possible.
- Unfortunately, all sort of things happen to students that can interfere with their studies. Lecturers and academic staff are very knowledgeable and sensitive to student experiences (we were once students and some of us still are!) If you anticipate that you may not submit your assignment on time please inform your tutor.
- Advise your families of your assignment submission date. If your family knows why you are working extra hard, you are more likely to get some help with housework and childcare (see Chapter 2).

## Stage 3: The Writing Phase

- As you begin to write down your notes and ideas, you will feel less anxious and your jotting will become more meaningful.
- As your assignment takes shape, your confidence will increase. Again we stress the importance of using your tutorial time to discuss any difficulties and questions you may have. We can promise you that you will not be alone!
- People write in different ways. For example, we find using headings and sub-headings an effective way of outlining an assignment. We can then add relevant key points in each section and slowly the assignment is constructed.  As you have already organised the literature, this task will be quite straightforward.
- Some people write straight to the computer, others write by hand and then to the computer. Overall, we would recommend draft form first and then the computer; this two-stage process allows for editing as you transfer your work to the computer. Indeed, you may have to write at least one draft before you are satisfied with the final result.

Once the draft has been achieved you can apply a spell-check and a grammar-check from your word-processing software but do not rely on them as they are fallible. For example, a word-processing spell-check will not pick up the word 'form' which is a misspelling of the word 'from'. Software packages do not replace reading the project yourself for spelling and grammar checks. When you have completed these you are ready for your first printout of your full project, but this will need further work so do not be under the illusion that you have finished – you haven't! You now need to undertake recension, which means re-reading the manuscript to correct any mistakes. This is of vital importance and cannot be stressed enough. Re-read your assignment from start to finish again and ensure that it makes sense, that there are no spelling mistakes, that the grammar is correct and any jargon has been removed. Make any changes that you wish to and check that your sub-heading structure remains intact and consistent.

## Learning Aid

**Assignment Check List**

| Assignment Activity | Date Commenced | Date Completed | Assignment Comments (eg. Appointment with tutor, any difficulties, library visits, etc.) |
|---|---|---|---|
| Literature Search | | | |
| Title | | | |
| Abstract | | | |
| Introduction | | | |
| Literature Review | | | |
| Discussion | | | |
| Conclusion | | | |
| References | | | |
| Printing, Binding | | | |
| Submission | | | |

This is a standard assignment brief. Of course, other assignments, particularly research studies, may have different headings and these can be changed accordingly. Students who find the prospect of writing a 3,000 word essay daunting, may find that writing a small amount every day and ticking the appropriate box when completed is a much more comfortable experience, and they will be pleasantly surprised to see how fast the assignment is completed!

## Learning Aid

Would the assignment make sense to someone else?
Can it be improved in any way?

# Peer Review

Depending on the type of project that you are submitting, you may now be in a position to have your work peer-reviewed. In doing assignments for course work you must produce work that is entirely your own and any collusion may be considered plagiarism. However, in writing for publication, constructing reports and presenting theses then it may be appropriate to ask a colleague to read your work for a critical appraisal. Check with your course organisers or supervisor before doing so, in order that you do not contravene university or college regulations. If you are able to have your work peer-reviewed, ask a colleague who is at the required academic standing to read your work. They should read it and make any comments that are appropriate. When they have done this they may hand it back to you with 'red' pen marks all over it, so do not be alarmed. Take the comments with good grace and remember that they are suggestions only. They will be comments from another person's perspective and they may have found mistakes that you have missed. Go through the comments carefully and if you agree with them make any adjustments to your project that you think will improve the work. Having your work perused by others may make you feel vulnerable, but this process will improve your work immensely and make your finished project a more professional product. Finally, make the number of copies required for submission, and a spare, and ensure that they are presented with the correct type of cover or folder and with the correct type of spine, if needed.

## Peer Review?

Depends on type of project.
Check with course organisers.
Take critique in good spirit.

## Improving Your Marks

As you become more practised and confident in your writing, you will see that your marks will begin to improve and this will give you a greater incentive to work for better results. Whereas at the beginning of your course you were relieved with a pass, now you want a distinction! However, we often see students finding it difficult to attain the high marks they desire and once they have reached a certain point their results may level out. This can be frustrating, and students say things like: 'I've done everything I can but I've still only got 56 per cent. What more can I do?'

Once the assignment basics of answering the question, keeping to the word limits, using references appropriately and correctly, using headings and sub-headings, spelling and grammar have all been mastered it would seem fair that the student should be awarded 100 per cent! Alas, this is not the case! There are some well known areas of assignment writing that students do not always address and hence they miss out on those coveted marks. We will mention two areas that will help students raise their marks; critical thinking and its partner, critical analysis.

Many people argue that critical thinking is a fundamental prerequisite of professional nursing practice. However, conveying both critical thinking and critical analysis in writing can be quite a challenge.

---

## Box 5:10    Assignments That Demonstrate Critical Thinking and Critical Analysis

The Critical **DANCE**

| | |
|---|---|
| **D**ebates | Should be reasoned and all issues equally discussed |
| **A**nalysis | Of arguments should go through a process of de-construction and re-construction. |
| **N**ew | Themes from reasoned debates have the potential to emerge in the process of analysis |
| **C**ategorisation | Of the debate into themes are central to the critical analysis |
| **E**xpression | Of new ideas may further the debate. |

---

## Conclusions

Writing tends to cause many people some degree of discomfort. This is for at least two reasons: first, there is a set of rules for writing which involves correct spelling and correct sentence construction; second, when you write something down you make your inner thoughts 'visible' for others to see, and this in turn makes you feel vulnerable. However, modern-day computers mean that you can constantly change a sentence or paragraph until you are happy with the finished product. You need to remember that writing is like sculpting and you can craft a paragraph, manipulate it and mould it to your required shape. The single most important aid to producing a good piece of writing is to re-read constantly what you have written, sometimes quietly to yourself and sometimes out loud to an imaginary audience. Writing is a skill that needs to be learnt and, like many skills, the more you practise it the better you become.

> ## SUMMARY POINTS OF CHAPTER 5
>
> - Writing, particularly for new students, can be an uncomfortable experience that makes them feel exposed and vulnerable.
> - There are a number of important rules of writing that students need to be familiar with to incorporate into their own assignments and essays.
> - Avoidance strategies are common amongst all writers; there are ways in which these can be converted into rewards for writing.
> - Planning and identifying an appropriate structure for writing is crucial to ensure a successful outcome. Follow the assignment writing process.
> - The phenomena of 'writers' block' and the 'blank page' are real challenges which can be overcome by employing useful strategies.
> - Reading and re-reading work before it is submitted is a vital stage of the writing process, but one which is frequently overlooked.

## Test Your Study Skills ...

1. What is meant by recension? (see page 96)

2. What are the four basic types of writing style? (see page 83)

3. What is the main problem with writing personal accounts? (see page 83)

4. How would you overcome the fear of the blank page? (see page 87)

5. How would you plan to write a 3,000-word assignment to be presented in one month, given that you have read all the literature? (see pages 87–88)

6. What is the most effective way of undertaking a spell-check? (see page 96)

## Practical Session ...

1. Write down your five favourite avoidance strategies (see page 84).

2. Write down a basic heading and sub-heading structure for a research paper (see page 90).

3. Write down a heading and sub-heading structure for an official report (see page 92).

4. Draw a check-list table for your next assignment (see page 97).

# 6 Referencing

## Introduction

Many students, not just of nursing but from many areas of study, complain bitterly about references and referencing. These moans and groans range from an inability to understand the importance of referencing to accusations of pedantry, and from a lack of insight into the seriousness of missing central references to a blind belief that their 'system' is a better one! In this chapter we will try to dispel at least some of this 'fog' and provide you with not only a better understanding of why we reference, but also a practical guide on how to do it. We will also emphasise the importance of referencing accurately and the need to provide supportive evidence for statements that are made. Although there are many ways of referencing we can identify three main types, which we will briefly outline. However, as the Harvard system is the most commonly used in the UK we will examine this system more closely. Accurate referencing is important both in the text and in the reference list at the end of the assignment and we will explain how both these tasks are undertaken.

## The Importance of Referencing

In a broad sense, accurate referencing is important so that other students who follow a similar course of study can track down the sources and check that they are accurate. References are used to support an argument, to make a claim or to provide evidence. This occurs as much when undertaking nursing projects as it does when evidence is presented in court or in a learned journal in support of a new treatment intervention.

Although one may readily accept the importance of the latter two examples, in the former, undertaking nursing prospects, nurses are often less convinced. When we are reviewing the literature, as in Chapter 4, we are reading, interpreting and synthesising other people's work, and the conclusions that we are drawing from them must be open to scrutiny by others. Therefore, the referencing must be accurate in order that others can track it down and check our interpretation by their own reading of the material. We must not be afraid of other people's reading of the literature that we may be reviewing, as different interpretations are always helpful in confirming or refuting a particular idea. In this way knowledge grows, ideas expand and concepts are focused. Many an aspiring academic has come unstuck by inaccurate referencing.

A second reason why accurate referencing is important is because certain documents that nurses produce may become public documents. When you leave a gap in a reference (i.e. date, volume, pages, etc.) it indicates to the reader that the author is academically immature.

Master's theses and PhD theses, written by nurses, become accessible to the public through university libraries and can, themselves, be referenced. Therefore, the skill and expertise of accurate referencing should be learnt at an early stage in one's career. Furthermore, as we mentioned in Chapter 5, nurses are increasingly asked to become members of committees, boards or inquiries, and in the course of their duties these bodies are frequently requested to produce reports, policies or framework documents. These documents, again, may be accessed by other disciplines or by members of the public. Even those documents that are held in confidence, and are not subject to scrutiny by the public, may well become the focus of an inquiry or presented as evidence in court. Care plans, case conference reports, clinical notes and nursing process forms have all been scrutinised by courts of law at one time or another. Being called to account for an inaccurate reference in a court of law would be highly embarrassing and likely to be damaging both to one's career as well as to our profession. This brings us to the third level of importance.

## Learning Aid

How would it feel to be in the witness stand and be questioned regarding the quality of your written work? How would you feel if another witness suggested that you referenced your work poorly?

The third level of importance refers to a question of professionalism. All nurses write some form of documentation in the course of the shift, and we are moving ever closer to a time in which our practice must be evidence-based. This involves referencing writ large. Our colleagues in the related healthcare professions are, by and large, already used to this and appreciate the need for a professional approach when producing written material. To the skilled academic eye, either in our other healthcare disciplines or within the legal profession, the way in which references are used and reproduced will give an indication of the professional educational standing of the nurse-author. As we mentioned above, in the course of being university lecturers we often hear student nurses say that they 'don't want to write, they just want to nurse'. Be under no illusion that the days of nursing as a practical endeavour alone have well and truly passed, and we are now held accountable for our nursing actions via the written word. This involves referencing and, in short, it is a matter of professional principle.

## Learning Aid

Writing, and especially referencing, is likely to become ever more important and necessary in nursing. So, practise and make perfect.

Two final points are worthy of mention regarding the importance of referencing, although they may well be considered of minor consequence by some. The first concerns the 'missing' reference; that is, the reference that is quoted in the text but omitted from the reference list. Sometimes references are taken out in the editing stage and we therefore advise that students check that all the references in the final list are still included in the body of the text before submitting their work. It is highly irritating for those who wish to follow up a reference to find that it is not given at all, not given in full or is given inaccurately in the reference list. This, again, does not help the individual student, and in a small way, but in effect, fails to assist the development of the nursing profession. The second, and final, point refers to the respect that we ought to have for others' work. Someone has gone to a considerable amount of effort to publish an article or book and we should do them justice by referencing them appropriately and correctly. Who knows, we might be referencing you one day. Box 6:1 highlights the importance of referencing.

## Box 6:1    The Importance of Referencing

References are important because ...

- Others need to track down the evidence.
- They support an argument.
- They provide evidence.
- They are an indicator of quality work.

*(Continued)*

*(Continued)*

- They show a degree of professionalism.
- They are a courteous way of recognising others' work.
- They assist in avoiding plagiarism.

## Professionalism?

Avoid missing references.
It is courteous.

# When to Reference

The question of when to reference may sound a strange one, but many times students make statements in projects without providing a reference source, and are criticised for it or even have marks deducted. There are several rules which should be applied to written material, and the first concerns referencing other people's work. If you write other people's comments down verbatim (the exact words) and do not provide a reference, then you are guilty of plagiarism, and this is a serious matter indeed.

## Learning Aid

In many academic institutions plagiarism is considered to be so serious as to warrant instant failure and possibly expulsion.

If you are going to use others' written words then provide quotation marks and a reference. For example:

Burden (2001: 498) stated that 'providing a detailed review of the literature on a given topic often poses difficulties for the prospective writer'.

Note here that the quotation marks indicate that they are Burden's words and not ours. Also note that we have included the page number on which the words appeared in Burden's publication.

The second rule about when to reference concerns the production of evidence. If we are going to make a claim, say, that reviewing the literature is important for nurses, we can support this claim by citing a number of authors who have made this suggestion in general terms. For example; 'it is felt that nurses having the ability to review the literature properly is important (Green, Johnson and Adams, 2000; Lutters and Vogt, 2000)'.

Both these sets of authors have published articles in which they suggest that reviewing the literature is important but in this case the actual words are ours and in our opinion these authors would generally support our view according to our reading of their work. However, the articles themselves are, in fact, very different and deal with very different topics, so the referencing is only a generalised claim.

## Learning Aid

Do not use too general a reference and be sure that you do justice to the spirit of the author's point of view.

The third rule of referencing is concerned with the more specific, and grand, statements that students often make. For example, I may wish to make a comment on the poor quality of review papers in epidemiology. This would be fine unsupported if we were epidemiologists who had read all the review papers in epidemiology and had found them to be of a poor quality. In this case we could write, 'in our view the review papers in epidemiology are generally of a poor quality'. However, as neither of us are epidemiologists, nor have read all the review papers in epidemiology, we would need supporting references for the claim that the review papers are generally of a poor quality, for example '(Breslow, Ross and Weed, 1998). 'Box 6:2 shows when you should consider referencing.

## Box 6:2   When to Reference

Generally you should reference ...

- When you use someone else's words (i.e., in quotation marks).
- When you are making a claim.
- When you need to provide evidence.
- When you need support for a statement or point of view.
- When you provide a statistic or specific example.
- When you need a source for a theory.

## Types of Referencing

Journals and publishing houses may have different styles of referencing, and should you be sending a manuscript to them with the view to publishing your own work then you would need to check what their house style is before sending it. Publishing houses have booklets (usually called 'Guide for Authors') and journals publish their own guidelines periodically in their own journals. However, overall there are basically four types of referencing system. There are variations within these systems, so check which one is needed for a particular assignment. If you are allowed to choose, we suggest that you choose the Harvard system. Whichever one you do use, be consistent.

- **The Legal System.** This system is used extensively in legal circles and when authored by lawyers official reports may employ this approach. It entails the use of footnotes on the page, which will usually be in a smaller font size than the main text and may contain references and explanatory notes (see Box 6:3). The advantages of the use of the legal system are that the full references and notes are usually on the same page and do not need searching for, and they also provide all the relevant extra information that the author deems necessary. However, the main drawback is that when they are used extensively, as they often need to be in legal work, they can be cumbersome and break up the flow of the main text.

## Box 6:3   Legal System of Referencing

From many philosophical works the theme of individualism features large.[1] Within this framework[2] there are numerous variants but all carry one central feature.[3] There are both negative[4] and positive[5] aspects.

1. T. Mason, (1999) How to catch a cold: the art of managing protest. *Journal of Action Nursing*, 4(3): 17–28.
2. See also further works on philosophical frameworks which show how individualism may be thought of.
3. The central feature, which will be dealt with further below, is based on the notion of the self.
4. P. Tyler, (1997) Negative aspects of individualism. *Journal of Philosophical Nursing*, 17(4): 18–26.
5. D. Tench, (1998) How to view individualism from a positive viewpoint. *Philosophical Medics*, 12(6): 18–30.

- **The Vancouver System.** This system is widely used in many journals and books and is particularly popular with publishers in the US. The system employs numbers, usually in superscript, where the reference is needed. The numbers are then listed in numerical order at the back of the manuscript with the full reference. One number is used for a particular reference so that you can use the same number throughout the paper whenever that reference is needed (see Box 6:4). The main advantage of this system is that the numbers do not break up the flow of the text as much as authors' names in brackets tend to do if over-used. The main disadvantage is that it is often the case that names of authors can provide general information about a point that numbers do not provide without an annoying search through the list at the back of the manuscript.

---

## Box 6:4    Vancouver System of Referencing

**In Text**

From many philosophical works the theme of individualism features large.[1] Within this framework there are numerous variants but all carry one central feature. There are both negative and positive aspects.[2,3]

**In Reference List at Back**

1.  Mason, T. (1999) How to catch a cold: the art of managing protest. *Journal of Action Nursing*, 4(3): 17–28.
2.  Tyler, P. (1997) Negative aspects of individualism. *Journal of Philosophical Nursing*, 17(4): 18–26.
3.  Tench, D. (1998) How to view individualism from a positive viewpoint. *Philosophical Medics*, 12(6): 18–30.

---

- **The APA System.** In the social sciences it is common to employ the American Psychological Association (APA) guidelines on referencing style. This Association publishes a manual to show how referencing should be structured. The APA standardises this format and many journals insist that this style should be used. Although there are many acceptable ways of referencing, and many journals have slightly different house styles, the APA referencing system standardises the format according to their agreed structure. To set up an APA reference list see Box 6:5.

---

## Box 6:5    APA System of Referencing

**Books** – Author, Date, *Title of Book*. City: Publisher.
Example – Mason, T. (1999) *Cold Catching*. Liverpool: Mersey Publishing.

**Journal Article** – Author, Date, Title of journal article. *Title of Journal*. Volume number, (Issue number). page extent.

*(Continued)*

*(Continued)*

Example – Mason, T. (1999) How to catch a cold: the art of managing protest. *Journal of Action Nursing*. 4(3): 17–28.

**Chapter in Book** – Author, Date, Title of chapter. In Editor's initial and name, *Title of Book*, Page range of chapter, City: Publisher.
Example – Mason, T. (1999) Catching more than a cold. In E. Whitehead (ed.), *Studying Protests*, pp. 187–214. Liverpool: Mersey Publishing.

**Internet Document** – Author, Date, Title of electronic text, [e-text type], Location of document, Date accessed.
Example – Mason, T. (1999) Cold catching [web page] urllhttp://www.colds.org/aetiology.html. Accessed 17 April 2007

- **The Harvard System.** This system is more popular with British-based publishing sources and uses the names of authors and the year of publication either in the written text, or enclosed in brackets in the text. The main advantages and disadvantages are the reverse of those in the Vancouver system. That is, the use of authors' names provides a good source of information but they can break up the flow of reading, especially if used extensively. As this system is more popular in British journals and universities we will concentrate more on this system in the following section.

## Learning Aid

Study the Harvard system very closely as you will need to know this at some stage of your writing.
The main systems are Legal, Vancouver, Harvard and APA.
There are others.
There are variations within each one.

# How to Use the Harvard Referencing System

As we say above, each publisher and university may have a preferred style of referencing, even within the overall system of the Harvard. We know of several universities that allow the student to choose a system that suits them best, but do not allow the mixing of systems within a project. Other universities are more prescriptive and demand the use of one system only, so check before submitting any work. The Harvard system, like the Vancouver system, has two main components: (a) using references in the text and (b) constructing the reference list.

# Using References in the Text

As mentioned above, we can use references in two ways: as primary sources in which we are directly referring to what another author has written, or secondary sources in which we are indirectly referring to what someone else has stated. The first point that we will deal with is an elaboration on the direct quote mentioned above in the 'when to reference' section. Using direct quotes is a very helpful method of providing evidence or in stressing a point, and the general rules of using quotes are as follows.

## *Primary Sources*

- Use sparingly.
- Do not quote more than 400 words, as you will then require written permission from the publishers.
- Quotes of approximately 2–3 lines can be included in your sentence structure. Example:

  Occupational therapy is a fast developing field of study but Snider (2000: 5) asked, 'who really cares about evidence-based practice in occupational therapy?'

  Note Snider's question mark within the quotation marks. Also note that here we have included the author's name within our sentence structure and only put the year of publication and page number in the brackets. Another way of writing this could be as follows:

  Occupational therapy is a fast developing field of study but a question has been raised: 'who really cares about evidence-based practice in occupational therapy?' (Snider, 2000: 5).

  Note here that the author's name is not part of the sentence structure and is now placed at the end of the quote in brackets. Also note that our full stop comes at the end, after the brackets.

- If more than three lines of quotation are being used then the quote can begin on a new line and be indented and set as an extract. Example :

  Occupational therapy is a fast developing field of study but a question has been raised:

  > Who really cares about evidence-based practice in occupational therapy? Is it only meaningful to graduate students, academics or other people whose major preoccupation is jumping through academic hoops? I don't think so. (Snider, 2000: 5)

  Note that no quotation marks are needed, but this varies according to publishing house or university, so check the rules. The indented quote should be single line spacing, irrespective of what the spacing is in the main text and note the full colon, which precedes the quote.

- If part of the original quote is being left out, this is indicated by three dots (ellipsis). Example:

Occupational therapy is a fast developing field of study but a question has been raised: 'who really cares ... in occupational therapy?' (Snider, 2000: 5).

Note that the sequence is: space, ellipsis, space. Also note that by employing the ellipsis we have significantly altered Snider's original meaning, so take care not to do this by omitting vital words.

- If there is an emphasis in the original quote you leave it in and say so in brackets at the end of the quote. Example:
(emphasis in the original).

- If you wish to place an emphasis in someone else's quote then do so and say this in brackets at the end of the quote. Example:
(author's emphasis).

- If you are citing a reference that is mentioned in a book but you are not reading it yourself you must reference both in the text and list the book that you are actually reading. Example:

Cohen (1979, cited in Nachmias and Nachmias, 1981).

In this example you are reading the Nachmiases' book and they mention Cohen. Therefore, you put the Nachmiases' book in the reference list and mention both in the sentence that you are writing, as indicated in our example.

- If there are more than two authors then the first surname is given, followed by 'et al.', on its second usage. However, all authors should be cited in the reference list. If there are two authors, then both are cited throughout the text.

## Using Primary Sources?

Quote accurately.
For omitted words use ...
Give author, year and page number.
Use 'et al.' correctly.

Box 6:6 incorporates most of these examples.

## Box 6:6    Example of the Harvard Referencing System (references are fictitious)

It is felt that violence is on the increase (Smith, Brown and Turner, 1994; Wishart, 1996; Bladon et al., 2000). However, this statement has been challenged by others working in the field (Marsh, 1998; Nielson and Grubin, 2001). Furthermore, Williams (2002: 142) has claimed that 'whilst it would appear that violence has increased in our society the statistics do not support this and it is more likely to be the fact that communication of violence is better than it has ever been in our history'. This would suggest that modern-day communication systems inform the general public of violence, which historically we may not have been aware of. However, it has been pointed out 'we cannot avoid the fact that the increase in the use of illicit drugs has caused an *increase* in criminal activity ... and this has led to an *increase* in fear' (Fisher, 2001: 8) (emphasis in the original). It would seem fair to suggest that certain types of violence have increased whilst others have remained static. Yet, some feel that it is the fact that violence against certain vulnerable groups is causing the greatest concern:

> It matters less that football hooligans beat each other senseless, or that gangland leaders are at war with each other, than it does when the elderly, disabled, children or women get attacked. What we can say with confidence is that these *vulnerable* groups have never been so *threatened* in our society. (Bull and Gardner, 2002: 48) (author's emphasis)

Finally, we can focus on the issue that it certainly *feels* like violence is on the increase and as Bannerman (1979, cited in Jones, 1988: 19) noted, 'fear is real whether it is actual or imagined'. In conclusion, we can say that it is certainly believed that violence is on the increase (Smith et al., 1994).

## Learning Aid

Go to an academic book or journal and observe how the authors have referenced in the text. Are there too many or too few references?

### Secondary Sources

Secondary sources are used to show that we have read supporting evidence for certain points of view or for developing lines of argument. In the use of references as secondary sources we are employing them more generally and less specifically than in primary sources. Secondary sources have two distinct meanings in terms of referencing. First, they refer to one author's interpretation of another author's work. For example, we might find the original text of a philosophical author difficult to understand and look for someone else's interpretation of that work. In doing this we are employing a secondary source. Second, they refer to an indirect reference in support of a particular argument or statement. for example, Miller (1994) considered Michel Foucault's work to be profoundly original. This, of course, is rather weaker than a direct primary reference source but is certainly better than none at all. The use of secondary sources is often criticised as being more tenuous in terms of the relationship between a line of argument and a fully supportive reference.

## Learning Aid

Avoid too many secondary sources. Avoid writing what Smith said that Green believed about Brown's interpretation of Turner's work!

The rules for the use of secondary sources overlap with those for the primary sources but have a few distinct rules of their own because we can employ them differently.

- If we wish to write a general statement that has been made by a number of authors from different sources we can reference them all in brackets with each reference separated by a semi-colon. Example: (Smith, 1999; Green and Brown, 2000; Edwards et al., 2001). Note that they are ordered according to the year of publication.
- If there are too many references to use – and the student should beware of stating too many in one set of brackets as they become cumbersome and break up the flow of reading – then place 'for example' at the beginning of the brackets. Example: (for example, Smith, 1999; Green and Brown, 2000; Edwards et al., 2001).
- If one author, or the same authors, have produced more than one reference in the same year then these are differentiated by lower-case letters after the year of publication. Example: The first paper is referenced (Rogers, 1999a), the second paper (Rogers, 1999b) and the third paper (Rogers, 1999c), wherever necessary throughout the text. Remember that the letter denotes the actual paper so should only relate to that paper and these should correspond in the reference list.
- If one set of authors has produced papers or books in the same year and you wish to refer to them in one set of brackets, omit the names following the first citation. Example: (Rogers, 1999a; 1999b; 1999c).
- If using the same author but different years of publication in the same brackets then no letters are necessary. Example: (Rogers, 1999; 2000; 2001).

- If different authors of the same name have produced papers in the same year they are distinguished by the initial of their Christian name. Example: (E. Morrison, 2000; P. Morrison, 2000).
- If an old book is re-published then it carries both years of publication. Example: Hobbes, T. ([1651] 1976) *Leviathan*. Harmondsworth: Penguin. Note the employment of two types of brackets with the original year of publication placed in the first set of brackets and the current publication in the second set.

## Using Secondary Sources?

Support general statements.
Avoid using too many for one statement.
If different authors have the same surname and year of publication then use their initial letters.

## Learning Aid

Write to a publishing house and ask them for a copy of their 'Guide for Authors'. They are usually very helpful.

## Constructing the reference list

Many nurses do not appreciate the importance of accurately constructing the reference list at the end of the manuscript. To reiterate, it is important for a number of reasons. First, future students, not to mention lecturers, may wish to check the reference source; second, a set format is required by publishers; and third, it is a question of professionalism.

- **Reference for a complete book, single author.** Example: Lorig, K. (2000) *Patient Education: A Practical Approach*. London: Sage. Note where the comma, full stops and colon are placed. Note that the title of the book is emphasised, which can be by underlining or italicising but you must use the same style throughout the list; the book title also has capital letters. The main structure is: name of author, initial, year of publication, title of book, place of publication and publisher. There are variations on this depending on the publishing house but for your project the important thing is to remain consistent.
- **Multiple authors and the inclusion of an edition.** Example — Roper, N., Logan, W.W. and Tierney, A.J. (1996) *The Elements of Nursing: A Model for Nursing Based on a*

*Model of Living* (4th edn). London: Churchill Livingstone. Take careful note of the commas, full stops and colon, as well as the insertion of the edition. This format is used for two or more authors with the 'and' inserted between the two authors if there are only two and between the last two for multiple authors.

- **Journal article.** Example: Andrews, M.M. (1999) How to search for information on transcultural nursing and health subjects: Internet and CD-ROM sources. *Journal of Transcultural Nursing*, 10(1): 69–74. Note that the journal has capital letters and is emphasised. The numbers following the journal refer to the volume, the part or issue (in the brackets), and the page numbers (after the colon). Multiple authors are listed as in the book reference.
- **Chapter in an edited book.** Example: Campbell, P. (1998) Listening to clients. In P.J. Barker and B. Davidson (eds), *Ethical Strife*. London: Arnold. The structure of this is: the author of the chapter (Campbell), the year of publication (1998), the title of the chapter (Listening to clients), the editors (Barker and Davidson), the name of the book (*Ethical Strife*), the place of publication (London) and the publisher (Arnold). Note that the book is emphasised and not the title of the chapter. Also note that the initials of the editors come before their surname.

## Referencing Other Source Material

Although books and journal articles are the main sources for references there are a number of other sources that are increasingly being used:

- **Unpublished material such as theses, pamphlets, leaflets, etc.** Example: Jones, J.J. (1997) Nursing Action in Accident and Emergency. PhD thesis, Manchester University, unpublished. Note that the structure is author, year of publication, title of work, what it is, whose property it is and its unpublished status.
- **Newspaper articles.** Example: *The Times* (1996) Scientists Attempt Cloning, international news report, 1 April. Note that in this case the newspaper is named as the author as occasionally newspaper articles do not carry an author's name. However, if an author is given, as in a special feature, then it is acceptable to put their name at the beginning of the reference and put the name of the newspaper between the international news report and the date, and then put the page number last. Example: Smith, J. (1996) Scientists Attempt Cloning, international news report, *The Times*, 1 April, p. 4.
- **Government and official publications.** Example – Cabinet Office (1991) *The Citizen's Charter: Raising the Standard*, Cmnd 1599, London: HMSO. The structure here is the government department source, the year of publication, the title, the command number, the place where the department is and the publisher.

- **Videos.** Example — *Managing Violence* (2000) Produced by Mark Sully and directed by Bob Parsons. 28 mins. North West NHS Trust Video Unit. Videocassette. Note the structure is the title of the recording, which is italicised, year of production, producer and director, duration of the video, details of the production unit and type of recording.
- **Houses of Parliament:** Example: *Hansard* (1992) Vol. 1054, cols 79–82. London: HMSO. Note the structure here is the official report of proceedings (*Hansard*), year of proceedings (1992), volume, columns, place and publisher.
- **Internet.** Example: *Health Care Funding Sources* (1999) Names and addresses. www.hcfs.gov/names.addresses.htm (accessed 4 April 1999). Note here that the structure changes to the broad source, the year, the specific source, the web address and when it was accessed.

## Conclusions

The use of references in a written piece of work is a reflection of scholarly quality and should be undertaken carefully and diligently. Good referencing in the text reveals depth of reading around the topic and gives an indication of the writer's knowledge of the issues. The reference list should be accurate, complete and standardised for style. Finally, as we have mentioned several times, but would like to reiterate once more, each publisher and university may have their own preferred house style, so find out what they want and give it to them.

---

### SUMMARY POINTS OF CHAPTER 6

- Accurate referencing is a fundamental prerequisite of any piece of academic writing.
- Referencing provides supportive evidence for statements that are made.
- There are four types of referencing: Harvard, Vancouver, Legal and APA.
- The Harvard referencing system is the most commonly used in higher education.
- Students must be familiar with the Harvard referencing system, discussed in this chapter.
- An important part of learning about referencing is when and how to reference.

## Test Your Study Skills ...

1. What must you consider when using the Harvard referencing system? (see pages 108–110)

2. What significance is placed upon the reference list? (see page 113)

3. What is a secondary citation? (see pages 111–112)

4. How do you reference a book chapter? (see page 113)

5. How do you reference the material sourced from the internet? (see page 115)

6. How do you reference an official report? (see page 115)

## Practical Session ...

1. Obtain a copy of the referencing guidelines for your programme of study.

2. Practise your referencing technique, using a wide range of sources.

3. Check with your personal tutor that your work is correctly referenced.

# 7 Passing Examinations and Other Theoretical Assessments

## LEARNING OUTCOMES

1. To understand the significance of examinations in assessing students' academic performance in nursing studies.
2. To be able to identify personal strengths and weaknesses in preparing for examinations.
3. To work towards correcting personal limitations in a proactive manner.
4. To become familiar with the examination rules and regulations of the institution of study.
5. To understand the significance of developing a 'reservoir' of knowledge.
6. To take time to learn your strengths and weaknesses.

## Introduction

Part of the studying process involves preparation for examinations, which are, as we point out below, a necessary evil. For the vast majority of students, exams cause fear, anxiety and tension, and in this chapter we will discuss ways in which the student can prepare for exams and which will contribute to a reduction in this anxiety. We will offer guidance in understanding the rules and regulations of exams and how to 'navigate' the immediate time before, during and after the exam. Unfortunately, a small number of students are not successful at the first attempt in a particular exam and we will discuss how the student can learn to cope with the disappointment and prepare for a re-sit.

## Exams: A Necessary Evil?

One of the questions most frequently asked by students who study nursing is: 'Why should we have to take exams, when all we want to do is care for sick people?' This is usually born out of apprehension of the exam, rather than based on a logical reasoning process, as we are all very aware of the necessity of exams. However, for those who are not convinced we can put forward a number of very sound reasons why students of nursing should take exams, and these are as follows. First, we have already discussed in Chapter 1 the implications for all students studying in an institute of higher education. It is in this learning environment that students must meet the academic standards and rigour of their institution of study. Second, these academic standards are replicated by the professional body for nursing: the NMC. Third, the reasons why nursing students are required to take examinations are the same as for all other students. Examinations allow course organisers to assess how much of the course work students have understood and can recall when needed. Fourth, examinations are a very specific tool of scholarship that encourages students to learn in an energised and focused way. Finally, nurses are dealing with vulnerable people who are in some form of ill health, and applying care in these circumstances requires skill, expertise and competence. Would anyone really wish to be cared for by someone who had not been examined as to their ability to perform such a task?

We appreciate that many students may not have taken exams for a very long time and that this group of people are naturally very anxious about the prospect of taking them. To these students we advocate that they read the whole of this chapter and follow the sections on 'testing your study skills' and the 'practical session' very carefully. We know that other students may feel fairly confident about exams, particularly if they have just finished school or a college course where exams were an essential component. These students may wish to use the chapter to refresh their memories on certain aspects of the examination process. What is your experience of taking examinations? Use this chapter according to your experience and confidence.

We are both mindful and sympathetic to those students who have had poor experiences of exams, either because of 'nerves' or of failure. In this chapter we aim to demystify the 'world' of examinations and provide practical suggestions on how to achieve success.

## Learning Aid

Do not let bad experiences of past examinations cloud your present progress. Start afresh!

## Types of Theoretical Assessments

It is generally agreed that the traditional two types of theoretical assessments have been the examination and the essay (assignment). However, some courses have also engaged with various types of 'practical' assessments, such as being assessed on taking a case history or performing a particular clinical procedure. During your nursing programme you will become familiar with a number of different theoretical assessments that your creative lecturers will employ to test your knowledge and comprehension of a particular subject or speciality! Here is a brief overview of some of the most commonly used theoretical assessments:

## Unseen Examination

This remains one of the most common forms of assessment and it is also the one that causes the greatest anxiety. The purpose of the unseen examination is to test students' ability to draw upon a reservoir of knowledge that they have learnt in preparation for the exam. We will discuss the preparation and the exam itself throughout this chapter.

## Seen Examination

Students required to sit a seen examination are given the paper in advance of the exam. They are allowed to prepare for their exam over a period of time and this requires researching at a greater depth than for the unseen exam. The seen examination may sound easier, but students are expected to produce a more detailed and analytical examination answer.

## Assignment

An assignment is a set task, which normally incorporates a number of sub-components – for example, collecting and synthesising literature, discussion and debate of a given subject and the identification of conclusions. It usually takes the form of an essay, with a set wordage and presented in an academic style (see Chapter 5).

## Portfolio

This is a body of work that is put together by the student over a period of time. It can comprise varying materials that demonstrate the student's progress. The portfolio frequently includes a significant section on students' reflection (see Chapter 10). Portfolios are often a record of the student's placement. Portfolios may include such information as written work, diaries, reflections, demographic data, CV, and details of clinical work placements.

## Objective Structured Clinical Examinations (OSCEs)

Objective Structured Clinical Examinations (OSCEs) are practical examinations which assess practical skills that students are expected to demonstrate with skill and professionalism. The Skills Laboratory (for those students returning to nursing you can equate the Skills Lab with your memories of the classroom ward where we practised giving injections into an orange and passing naso-gastric tubes on each other!), is now a familiar, necessary and significant part of the student learning experience, where students can practise their skills under careful supervision in an environment which is safe and friendly. Blood pressure recording is an example of one of the skills which students are assessed on under the OSCE system.

## Case History

The case history, after some years in the 'wilderness', is now back in favour, and it is not difficult to see why it is once again popular. In this assessment, students are required to make a study of one patient/client under their care. The assessment is usually in the form of an assignment, but it may be an oral presentation. Students are expected to know in depth their patient's condition, treatment and care. They are normally also asked to discuss the social and psychological aspects of their care, providing a complete and holistic case history.

## Group Work

Group work, if used, is usually one part of a module assessment. It often involves at least two students working together on one project and presenting their work to the class, with their lecturer and a colleague marking their work. Seminars demonstrate students' ability to work together, but also to be able to present their work individually. There is a degree of pressure placed upon each student not to 'let the side down'! Marking may be of each student's own contribution or of the group as a whole.

## Poster Presentation

Poster presentations are visual assessments which allow students to demonstrate their skills in presenting their project or study in a creative and informative manner. Poster presentations vary from the strictly academic format to the more magazine-like arrangement. The type of poster used depends upon the project. For example, an empirical research study to be presented in poster form at an academic conference will take the form of a research article, including data collection, analysis, findings and discussion, etc. However, a poster to show the importance of healthy eating to primary school children will be somewhat different! In the latter instance students will be expected to deliver clear messages in an attractive form that children can understand.

## Video/Tape Recordings

Occasionally, students will be required to use video or tape recordings as part or whole of their assessments. This may be in the form of an interview, perhaps with students taking on the roles of the client and the professional. They are often used to demonstrate the student's appreciation and understanding of a particular situation and how they would react to certain events and address particular problems.

## Dissertation

The dissertation is normally one of the final pieces of work that students are expected to submit at the end of their programme of study, whether this is at undergraduate or post-graduate level. The wordage is usually up to three times as long as the assignments which they have been used to on their course. Frequently (particularly at Master's level) the dissertation will take the form of a research study which the student has devised, carried out and written up. At this point we would remind students to work closely with their supervisors and attend their tutorials. Dissertations are substantial pieces of work, carrying the proportionate number of marks, and students need to bring all their study skills to the fore!

## Thesis

We imagine most students reading this book will be new to nursing studies and therefore it is understandable that the idea of one day embarking upon an 80,000 word PhD (Doctor of Philosophy) thesis is unthinkable! Let us remind you that most of us start off with these sentiments. We remind ourselves that you are the university lecturers and researchers of tomorrow and we plant the seed here. Your generation will be the one where nearly every nursing lecturer carries the title of Dr – it could be you, yes you and you…

## Preparing for Examinations

Taking time to prepare for examinations is a crucial activity in achieving a successful outcome. Start by imagining being successful and avoid defeatist thinking. Illustration 7:1 reminds students of the domains of activities that have to be taken into account when preparing for their exams.

We will now address each of the issues raised in Illustration 7:1.

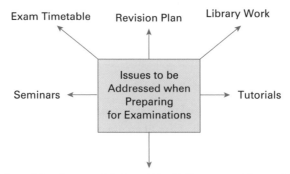

Organising Responsibilities of Family/Partner and Home Life

**Illustration 7:1   Areas to organise when preparing for examinations**

## Exam Timetable

Obtain your exam timetable as soon as possible; this will help you organise all your other responsibilities. Students will be given a timetable at the beginning of each new module. The module leader will explain the module handbook and discuss all the assignments and examinations. We suggest that students add these dates to their study plans and inform their families/partners as soon as possible, as it is important that all other activities be organised around both the exam and the revision for the exam.

## Revision Plan

We suggest that students set up a revision plan with realistic goals. Successful revision is a major part of studying and we discuss revising more fully in the section below.

## Library Work

Library work is required to extend and deepen a student's knowledge of any given subject, but this takes time and should not be left to the last minute. We suggest that students get into the habit of using the library regularly throughout the course of their study.

## Learning Aid

Students who do not use the library, or do so infrequently, do not have up-to-date supporting data for their written assessments and subsequently are unlikely to achieve high marks.

## Tutorials

We suggest that students arrange to see their personal/academic tutors well in advance of their examinations. A pre-examination tutorial allows students to discuss their anxieties and queries about any aspect of the exam and possibly get advice regarding areas for revision or weaknesses to be addressed.

## Seminars

Many schools and departments of nursing and midwifery run pre-examination seminars. Indeed, staff are usually quite willing to organise lunchtime seminars on exam technique, particularly if they are approached by students. We suggest that you enquire about them and make every effort to attend.

## Organising Responsibilities of Family/Partner and Home Life

We have discussed in a previous chapter the significance of communicating with families and partners about all aspects of the course. It is important that students give themselves the best possible chance of passing their examinations and, to help achieve this outcome, some students may need to organise additional care for any dependent relatives. Further planning is needed to organise family commitments, housework, shopping, and so on.

## Learning Aid

How much planning can I do before my exam? Have I covered all the domains of activity in this section?

If students are having problems organising their home life to fit into their examinations, we suggest that they see their personal tutors and the college student support services who may offer constructive help and advice.

## Revision

Revision means to take a fresh look at something that you have previously considered, and involves many strategies to ensure that you are able to recall the material that is required to show an examiner that you have the correct level of knowledge. Revision is not necessarily a question of memorising vast tracts of information but has more to do with constructing summaries and bullet points of what you have learnt about a particular topic. The importance of revision is only surpassed by the importance of doing it correctly. There is nothing so counter-productive as revising badly, as this is even worse than not doing revision at all. It is an active process that requires careful planning and systematic application in order for it to be effective. It is not a question of haphazardly reading through course notes, books and journals and hoping that something will 'stick' and that you will remember something for the exam. Therefore, you need to approach revision as a set procedure that has to be undertaken in a logical sequence of steps.

## Planning your Revision

The first step is to plan your revision. Ideally revision should start at the beginning of your course of study and you should revise the lecture, the paper, the book, the seminar, the module, and so on, as you go along. You should have a weekly revision plan in which you can revise the material that you have covered in that week. This can be followed by a monthly revision plan covering the month's work and a module or semester revision plan covering that material. This can be done year on year until your final exams.

---

### Learning Aid

Make a revision plan that incorporates all areas of your course and is geared towards a regular time frame.

---

Remember the 'reservoir' of knowledge mentioned in Chapter 1; if you have filled this 'reservoir' with information then you will have it available to draw on both for your revision and your exams. Revision is about going back over material that you have covered and is *not* about learning new information. Therefore, the revision plan should systematically cover what your course curriculum has outlined.

Not all students undertake revision throughout the course and some wait until the exam is upon them before they think about revision. In this situation the timing of the revision is very much a personal decision and you should think carefully about this. Some students leave it until the last couple of weeks before the exam to start their revision and others will use the last three months to revise. There are advantages and disadvantages to both, as you may not have enough time in the former and peak too soon in the latter. This is entirely your decision and will depend on your personal commitments in life, the time you have available for revising, your style of revision, the extent of your knowledge, and your personal goals on the course.

## Learning Aid

When making your decision to revise, make sure the factors that you are considering are genuine ones and not merely avoidance strategies.

Box 7:1 outlines some of the major decision factors that you should consider when you are timing and constructing your revision plan. Panic revision is bad revision, as it causes confusion and can make things worse for you. Therefore, the central point is to plan your revision appropriately and well in advance.

## Box 7:1   Major Decision Factors for a Revision Plan

- **Personal Commitments** — These involve your partner, children, family, friends, work, hobbies, and so on. You must get the balance right so that you are both committed to your revision and have commitment from others. Reward both yourself and others after the exam.
- **Style of Revision** — Think carefully about how you do revision. Are you a fast or slow writer? Do you like to revise out loud or quietly to yourself? These factors will determine whether you need to be alone or not.
- **Time Available** — There are two imponderables. There are only 24 hours in a day. The day of the exam will arrive. What you need to consider is how much time you have available, given all your other commitments, and how much time you need for your revision. A simple equation but a crucial one. Some things will need to be postponed and you may need to negotiate this.
- **Extent of Knowledge** — Assess how much knowledge you have in relation to the course, and gear your revision plan accordingly. Be realistic about how much knowledge you think you have. Don't be overconfident, but don't be underconfident either. You may feel that your mind is empty, but this is (usually) an illusion.
- **Personal Goals** — You will have your own set of goals in your course, and your revision will need to reflect this. If you are working towards a first-class honours (or equivalent), then clearly you will need to do more revising than if you just want a third-class pass.

## Doing Revision?

Make a revision plan.

The 'reservoir' must be filled.

The timing of revision is up to you.

Make time available.

## Some Revision Methods

The next step to undertake is to re-read all material, especially your course notes, and summarise modules, chapters, lectures, etc., into short bullet points. If you can make the bullet points very short, one or two words is ideal, then you can fit them onto one side of an index card (as shown in Chapter 4). Use one card for one topic and build them up until you have a series of cards for the entire curriculum. You can do this during the course as you progress through the content, which means that you do not have to undertake it when it is time for revision. However, if you do leave it until the revision time, then it is still a crucial exercise to undertake, as it is part of the revision process. Summarising is important as it establishes mental links between large amounts of information and simple trigger words, known as acronyms.

The next step is to formulate acronyms whenever you can and where it is appropriate. An acronym is a word with each letter representing another word. They can be useful memory prompts and help you to link into information at that point when panic is setting in and you think that you cannot answer a particular question. Take a look at the example of an acronym in Box 7:2.

## Box 7:2    Information Links of an Acronym

Breathing — Anatomy and physiology, obstructed breathing, nursing care of breathing difficulties, maintaining airway, conditions that cause breathing difficulties, equipment needed, drugs used, signs and symptoms, nebulisers, fear and anxiety, and so on ...

Eating

Drinking

Sleeping

Pain

Anxiety

Wound

Skin

We can see in the acronym BEDS that each letter links into a word; in our example the letter B stands for Breathing. The word 'breathing' then links into the many areas that are related to the respiratory tract, and also includes the fear and anxiety of having a breathing difficulty. The numerous areas that we have outlined are by no means exhaustive and you could possibly add many more. The important points to note are two-fold. First, that the 'reservoir' is 'filled' with knowledge of 'breathing'. Your course and training is about filling this 'reservoir', and hopefully you have read everything that you could, listened, experimented, questioned, challenged, thought and learnt throughout. If this 'reservoir' has been filled you can now draw on it. The second point is that as you approach the exam you tend to feel that your knowledge is negligible and insufficient to pass the exams. However, this is usually a false impression, especially if you have filled the 'reservoir', and what is more likely to be the case is that you have vast tracts of knowledge but you just feel that you cannot recall it at the moment. Therefore, what you are taking into the exams, at a conscious level, are merely a few acronyms.

## Learning Aid

What could you say about the 'E' in the acronym BEDS in Box 7:2?

Once you have summarised all your work into a series of bullet points and acronyms, and produced these on index cards, you can take a few cards per day and revise them until you are satisfied that you can reproduce them accurately. Carry a few with you in your pocket, bag or rucksack and take every spare moment to pick one out and revise it. You may also wish to produce cards with questions on one side and the answers on the reverse, which can be used in the same way as the index cards as a revision strategy.

## Reading for Revision?

Re-read all material.
Summarise into one or two words.
Summarise onto index cards.
Formulate acronyms.

## Learning Aid

You are now grown up and being a swot is not 'uncool'.

The next stage is to practise 'chaining'. By 'chaining' we mean to be able to establish links both from the acronym into the 'reservoir' of knowledge and between the initial letters of the acronym and the exam question that you are answering. For example, Box 7:3 highlights the relationship between the question, the acronym and the answer.

---

## Box 7:3    Example of Relationship between Question, Acronym and Answer

Question — A 70-year-old man suffering with emphysema is admitted to a medical ward following a fall in which he sustained a laceration to his arm. Outline the nursing care that will be delivered.

Now highlight which of the following letters of the acronyms that you think would be important to mention in your answer.

Breathing — Anatomy and physiology, obstructed breathing, nursing care of breathing difficulties, maintaining airway, conditions that cause breathing difficulties, equipment needed, drugs used, signs and symptoms, nebulisers, fear and anxiety, and so on ...

Eating
Drinking
Sleeping
Pain
Anxiety
Wound
Skin

Of course there are more factors (and acronyms) that need to be incorporated and this is only a basic example.

---

Although this is a simple example, and is largely incomplete, it serves to show how you can build up the 'chains' from the acronym to the 'reservoir' of knowledge, which provides you with a wealth of information to answer your question. Also note that the example given is that for a physical condition at a basic level, but that acronyms can be developed for all types and levels of courses, and share the same principles of linking between the letters of the acronyms and the 'reservoir' of knowledge.

## Want to Recall Information?

Practise 'chaining'.
Establish links between acronym and 'reservoir'.
Revise a few index cards per day.

## Past Papers

The next point we would like to consider is the acquisition of past exam papers. This can be done formally by asking your tutors or course leaders, or writing to the Examination Board. Or, it can be done informally by asking senior students who have sat the exam for a copy of their paper. In any event, you must become proactive in getting hold of the past exam papers and this can often be better achieved in a group where each member can employ a different approach and try a different channel. Any exam papers acquired can then be shared amongst the group.

## Learning Aid

A group can be set up for the purposes of studying and can be used for sharing, debating, posing questions, supplying answers, testing and supporting each other. But do not lose sight of your individual needs for learning and revising. Studying in a group is fine as long as you are satisfying your own needs.

Past exam papers are excellent for providing you with a wealth of information concerning the exam standards, but if these cannot be acquired ask your tutors for a specimen exam paper or mock exam paper instead. Past exam papers, or specimen and mock papers, provide a rich source of information, and allow you to practice the main problems in sitting exams. First, you need to establish how many questions there are, both to choose from and that you need to answer. In some exams the number of questions are many and you are asked to answer only a few of them, and in others you may not be given any choice and are told to answer set ones. Second, you need to know the length of time that you have for the exam and the time to answer each question. This is crucial and will be expanded upon in the section on sitting exams. Third, you will need to know if the exam paper is divided into different parts that require different types of answers. For example, some exam papers are set in two parts in which you are asked for short answers in one part and longer essay types in another part. Other exams are multiple-choice in which you are merely asked to mark a box indicating your choice of answer. Fourth, you will need to know how the content of questions relates to the information that you have received on your course, and, more importantly, the information that you have in your head. This will give you a good indication of the amount and content of revision that is needed. Fifth, you will need to know the style of language that is used in the exam questions. Exam questions are very difficult to set and some considerable time and effort goes into getting the wording correct. Sixth, you can use the past exam papers as revision exercises. Make sure you follow the instructions as in the exam and keep to the timing. Ask a tutor to look over your practice answers, and check with your course notes and books. Box 7:4 summarises the use of past exam papers.

## Box 7:4  Summary of Use of Past Exam Papers

- Number of questions to choose from.
- Number of questions to be answered.
- Number of parts to the exam paper.
- Relationship between content of questions and your knowledge.
- Style of language used.
- Revision exercises.
- Analysing questions.

Finally, past exam question papers will give you the opportunity to practise analysing the questions. This is particularly important as you must answer the question correctly, or, no matter how brilliantly you write, you will fail. You need to understand what the question is actually getting at, so read it several times and highlight which are the most important words. See Box 7:5 as an example.

## Box 7:5  Highlighting Key Words of an Exam Question to Help Form your Answer

Mrs Davies is an *active lady aged 70 years*. She is admitted to the Accident and Emergency Department after tripping over her *pet dog and has sustained a fractured neck of femur and facial bruising*. Mrs Davies is a *widow with no relatives*, but she has *reliable and supportive neighbours*.
*Discuss* Mrs Davies's *immediate and long-term treatment and nursing care*.

## What Use are Past Exam Papers?

Number of questions to be answered.
Length of time available.
Structure of the exam.
Weighting of the marking.
Content of the questions.
Style of language used.
Practise answering the questions.
Practise analysing the questions.

Remember that the examiners do not put superfluous information into a question so each major item should be covered and dealt with in your answer.

## Improving your Writing Ability

Two final points will be mentioned. First, consider your writing ability and check this for speed and legibility. With the modern use of word-processing packages and computers we tend not to write as much as we did previously. This may have led to a reduction in speed and legibility. If you think that you are a little slower than expected then practise writing past exam papers, as we say above, and keep within the timing set by the paper. Write every day to ensure that your writing muscles are strengthened.

Furthermore, the greatest answer in the world cannot be passed if the examiner cannot read your writing, so improve your legibility as much as you can. The second point is to keep a positive attitude. There are lots of psychological pitfalls when approaching exams. Therefore, keep motivated and keep to your plan. Use every moment as wisely as you can and remember that the end of the exam will come with the words 'put your pens down', and you can look forward to rewarding both yourself and your family and friends.

## Answering the Question?

Read the questions several times.
Highlight key words.
Check your speed of writing and legibility.
Keep a positive attitude.
In your exam answers, speed and quantity are not substitutes for relevance and quality.

# Rules and Regulations of Examinations

For many students their previous experience of the rules and regulations of examinations belongs to their school days. There are indeed similarities between the exam systems of school and higher education, but there are also differences, and students are advised not to assume that the rules of school examinations necessarily apply to higher education. We therefore begin this section by suggesting to students that they learn as much as possible about the rules and regulations concerning the theoretical assessments of their programme of study.

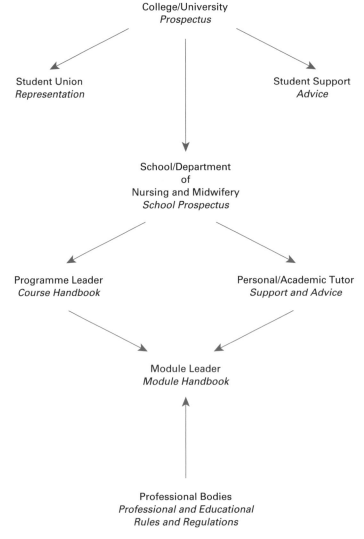

**Illustration 7:2   Accessing information on assessment rules and regulations within the college/university and professional body framework**

## Learning Aid

Plan ahead as much as you can, making time for exam revision.
Make sure that you obtain all the rules, regulations and assessment dates of your examinations as early as possible.

Illustration 7:2 provides students with the college framework of the examination structure and assessment information that can be obtained.

## Learning Aid

Exam results cannot be published within a few days. Students need to understand the marking system.

The process of marking is complex, involving second markers and external examiners. This ensures that the whole assessment procedure is conducted in a fair and ethical manner and that the academic and marking standards are maintained within the college. Box 7:6 shows students the stages of the marking process.

## Box 7:6   The Stages of the Marking Process

- **Stage 1** — Students submit assignments to the module leader and examination papers to the invigilator.
- **Stage 2** — The invigilator returns exam papers to the module leader (or examinations officer). Assignments are received by the module leader.
- **Stage 3** — The module leader distributes the assignments to academic tutors/module lecturing staff for 'first' marking.
- **Stage 4** — Markers return the marked papers within the stipulated time; this can vary but is usually one to three weeks.
- **Stage 5** — The module leader arranges a number of staff to 'second' mark a percentage of the papers; this will include a cross-range of marks, including all those students who have been awarded a 'fail'. Again the period given for 'second' marking varies but is usually about a week.

*(Continued)*

*(Continued)*

- **Stage 6** — The 'second' markers return the marked papers to the module leader.
- **Stage 7** — A number of institutions hold a 'mediation day' where all the assessments and examinations of a particular module are re-read. The weakest and the strongest work are given particular consideration.
- **Stage 8** — The module leader arranges (usually with the school/department examination officer) to send a percentage of the papers to the external examiner (see Box 7:7 for the role of the external examiner).
- **Stage 9** — The external examiner is sent a representative selection of all the scripts; this includes the highest marks, lowest marks (including all 'fails') and the middle marks. The external examiner is usually allowed two to three weeks (this can vary) to mark the work.
- **Stage 10** — The external examiner attends the examination or assessment board, which is usually held twice a year (this may vary depending upon assessment times and course intakes), delivers a report and confirms or ratifies the examination results. Alternatively she/he may require discussion or clarification before they sign the assessment mark sheets.
- **Stage 11** — The results are entered onto the students' files.
- **Stage 12** — The students are informed of the results. The usual procedure involves those students who have failed receiving letters of the result along with a request to contact their personal tutors, and those students who have passed having their results posted on the students' notice board.
- **Stage 13** — All those students who have unfortunately failed their theoretical assessments are seen individually and their future is discussed, taking into account their personal situation; for example, whether this failure has been a first or second attempt. Coping with setbacks is discussed in the last section of this chapter.

The external examiner is a crucial member of the assessment team. External examiners are required by every department/school within the college to ensure academic standards and rigour is maintained within every programme and module of study. Box 7:7 informs students of the role of the external examiner.

## Box 7:7    The Role of the External Examiner

- The appointment of external examiners is a mandatory requirement for all courses of study in higher education.
- External examiners are specialists in their field of study for which they have been appointed.

*(Continued)*

- External examiners are academic members of staff employed by institutes of higher education, for example, lecturers, senior lecturers and professors.
- External examiners are appointed for three years with an option to carry on for four years.
- Their practical role involves checking the marking of work by internal examiners for particular modules, attending examination boards and submitting annual reports.
- External examiners provide a crucial service and work in the interests of the school and the students. This is achieved by looking at the course of study as a whole as well as the particular components of assessment. The external examiner makes herself/himself familiar with the course; they check that students are examined on those subjects that are within the module content. They also check examination questions for parity and fairness before they are published. External examiners mark papers and check that the internal examiners have shown fairness and parity for each assessment and examination.
- External examiners are also called upon to adjudicate if there is a disparity of marks awarded by two internal examiners to one student.
- Some institutions, usually universities, employ the assessment of the viva voce or oral examination, to establish a degree classification. Viva voce is usually used when the classification is unclear, usually between a first-class honours degree and an upper second (2:1). On these occasions the external examiner will be asked to participate in an interview which asks the student a number of searching questions, allowing the student to demonstrate their knowledge.
- The advice of the external examiner is also sought in relation to those students who present particular challenges, for example, through illness or family issues that have caused or prompted them to fail their assessments.
- As practising academic lecturers in other institutes of higher education, external examiners are well placed to offer support and suggestions on all aspects of the assessment process.

In our experience, students present with a number of standard questions relating to the rules and regulations of theoretical assessments; for example: 'What happens if I'm sick on the day of the exam?' or 'What can I take into the exam?' These and other questions have been anticipated and incorporated in the following two sections.

## Submitting Assignments

The continuous assessment process, whereby students submit assignments to fulfil the theoretical requirements of particular modules, is for many students (depending upon their course structure) a more likely experience than the examination system. We suggest that students read Chapter 5 on Assignment Writing in conjunction with this section. There are a number of rules and regulations relating specifically to assignment writing, which students must be familiar with and these are bulleted as follows:

- Module leaders will have an assignment 'launch' date, when the details and submission dates of the assignment will be announced. Ensure you have these details and enter them in your diary.
- If you do not submit your assignment on the required date, assume it will be marked as a failed first attempt. If you have an emergency at home and cannot arrange for a colleague to submit your work on your behalf, you must telephone your module leader or personal tutor and explain the situation, before and *not* after the submission time.
- Ensure you follow all the rules of format for your assignment. For example, line spacing, font size and font style. These requirements are found in your programme handbook.
- Check your word count. The general rule is that candidates may write 10 per cent more or less than the stipulated number of words; any deviation from this and students must expect to have marks deducted.
- Ensure that all details asked for are entered on your assignment submission form; for example, full title of module and student number.
- Ensure you submit the required number of copies (and keep one for yourself!).
- If you are sick and cannot submit your work, you must inform your tutor and produce a medical certificate from your general practitioner. If you do not have a sick note, assume you will be marked as a failed attempt.

Students frequently expect to have their assessments marked and returned within a few days, which is unrealistic and should not be expected. If you plan carefully you will not be in a position where you are needing your assignments back urgently, so plan well ahead and hand your project in as soon as you are ready.

## Learning Aid

Students frequently overestimate the time they have available to write their assignments and consequently 'have' to see their tutors when it's too late and they are struggling to submit on time.

## Sitting Examinations

We have addressed this part of the 'passing exam' process by breaking this section into three sub-sections. First, preparing for the exam; second, the day of the exam; and, finally, after the exam. Students have different approaches to preparing for exams.

## Box 7:8    Preparing for your Examination

- Ensure you have an examination timetable. The timetables are posted on the student notice boards. Ensure you write down the examination dates, subjects, codes, time and duration, and location.
- Obtain a map of the college/university campus and visit the examination hall(s) before the day of the exam. Students who don't find their exam hall in advance frequently run around the campus on the day of the exam, panicked and late!
- Ensure you buy all the equipment you need for the exam and any special requirements; for example, if you are taking the Nursing Prescribing exam, you may need to buy a copy of the British National Formulary.
- Read the section on 'revision'. Organise your revision as soon as possible.
- We suggest a family meeting, to inform the members of your household of the exam dates and how this will affect them. We suggest that you ask your family to take on some of your commitments around the exams and the exam days. This will help you concentrate and focus your mind on the exams.
- We suggest that students reduce their paid employment as much as possible in the period before the exams.
- Adequate sleep, rest, exercise and a well-balanced diet will help students in their exam preparation and performance.
- If students have special educational needs, they must inform their personal tutor and module leader. For example, students with dyslexia may require extra time and coloured paper to write on. In some institutions the student and exams department will arrange additional facilities and invigilators. We also suggest that students contact the student support service who can offer practical and sympathetic help.

## Preparing for the Exam

In Box 7:8 we offer guidance on how students can prepare for their exams and we emphasise that students must plan around the revision and the exam, and must ensure that their other responsibilities have been covered. Negotiate help early and plan to reward those who have assisted you. Make sure that you pack the things you will need for the exam the night before and make sure that you have back-up pens and pencils. You may be able to take water and sweets into the exam, so make sure that these are packed in your bag, and do not take too many.

## The Day of the Exam

The day of the examination can be a very anxious time for students. Rise early in the morning and have a bath/shower. Try to eat some breakfast but make it a snack rather than a full meal. Remember that 'nerves' will make you want to visit the 'loo' a lot so make sure that you know where the washrooms are located and carry some tissues with you. Make sure that you leave plenty of time for travelling to the place of the exam and remember that if it can go wrong, it is highly likely to do so. Get an earlier train or bus than usual, and if you are using a taxi book it the day before and let them know that you are attending an exam and its importance to you. Give the taxi firm a reminder call in the morning.

In Box 7:9 we help students plan their exam day and anticipate some of the things that we know can happen unexpectedly!

## Box 7:9   The Examination Day Checklist

- Care organised for children/other dependent relatives.
- Transport organised (bus/train timetables, car with petrol in!).
- Enough money for day: fares, lunch.
- All requirements for exam: pens, pencils (and back-ups) and additional items as required.
- Map of campus, with exam hall highlighted.
- Copy of exam timetable.
- Student number (if appropriate).
- Additional personal items as required — keep these to a minimum, as you will be asked to leave your personal effects at the door of the examination hall.
- If you are sick on the day of the exam you must inform your personal tutor or module leader and obtain a sick note from your GP.
- If you have an emergency at home, inform your personal tutor or module leader as soon as possible.

## Learning Aid

The examination day can be an anxious time; plan ahead to reduce stress levels, for everyone concerned, as much as possible.

Each institute of higher education gives students a list of rules that they must abide by during the examination. Box 7:10 informs students of the general rules; some institutes will vary these, depending upon the examination procedure and format. It is advisable that students read this list carefully as penalties for breaking rules can be high. Students must also be aware that in many institutes they may be sitting their exams with students from other schools and departments across the college/university.

## Box 7:10    General Rules for the Conduct of Students during Exams

- Many institutes do not allow candidates into the examination hall if they arrive late.
- Candidates are not allowed to leave the examination hall outside the specific times stated.
- Candidates are only allowed to take the items required for the exam to their exam seat. All other items are usually left at the door, so we advise you not to take any valuables such as mobile phones and credit cards.
- Mobile phones are frequently banned from examination halls; if they are allowed, obviously they must be switched off!
- Candidates must listen very carefully to the invigilators, who will give them information about the exam (see Box 7:12) and instruct them on the necessary form filling.
- Do not turn over your examination paper or start the exam until the invigilator tells you.
- Candidates will have read in their programme handbooks about plagiarism. This is a serious offence and can lead to very severe penalties and any student caught cheating should expect to be dealt with accordingly.
- Students must not talk during exams.
- Any student who requires help must raise their hand and wait for the invigilator.
- If a candidate requires to go to the toilet, they are escorted by one of the invigilators.
- Ensure you follow the invigilator's instructions and write your number on each sheet of your answer book.
- You must stop writing when told to do so by the invigilator.

The invigilator is a crucial person in the examination process. Box 7:11 informs the reader of the significant duties of the invigilator.

## Box 7:11    The Role of the Exam Invigilator

- Invigilators are recruited from the institute academic staff and doctoral students. Module leaders may act as invigilators.
- Invigilators ensure that the exam is conducted in a smooth and fair manner.
- They are responsible for the issuing and returning of seat numbers, examination papers and answer books.
- They conduct the examination, informing candidates when they can start and when they must finish.
- Invigilators ensure that the exam scripts are collected and returned to the student and exams department or directly to the module leaders.
- Invigilators deal with emergencies and queries from the candidates.
- In some examinations there may be a number of invigilators, depending upon the number of students, the length of time of the exam and the complexities of the exam.

There are a number of small but significant points to remember when answering examination questions and these have been included within Box 7:12.

## Box 7:12    Useful Tips for Answering Examination Questions

- Always spend the first few minutes of the exam by reading carefully the exam instructions. Note the number of questions to be answered within each section (if the paper is divided into parts) and calculate the time required for each question. Questions may be given different mark weightings and this should be made clear next to each question.
- Read the exam questions carefully and underline key words.
- Write legibly.
- Answer only what is asked. Students frequently write down everything they know but the examiner can only mark what has been asked.
- Avoid spending all your time on one question; you cannot be given more marks than the maximum allocated.
- When you have finished your exam, ensure your number is on each page of the answer book. If you have additional sheets, tie them securely to your book.

## Getting Ready to Submit and Sit?

Find out what they want and give it to them.
Preparation is all-important.
Know the rules and regulations.
Manage the anxiety.

## After the Exam

After the exam try to avoid the 'post-mortem' analysis, at least until the next day. It is very tempting to ask the other candidates 'what did you put down for the question on ...?' and then to compare that with what you can remember you actually wrote. This then leads to panic because you probably did not put the same thing down in your answer. Remember, they may be wrong, not you. Also try to avoid preparing yourself for failure with comments such as 'I have done really badly', 'I never revised that area' and 'I know I've failed.' These comments are never convincing, either to yourself or to others.

## Coping with Setbacks

This textbook is about working towards and developing successful study skills in nursing. We appreciate that for some students success is not going to be achieved at the first attempt. Failing an exam or assignment is undoubtedly a miserable experience, and there can be any number of reasons for doing so. Students express a variety of emotions, including blame of themselves and others, sadness, anger and frustration. Once students have aired these feelings, they can begin to look to the future and make plans, better ones than before, to prepare and re-sit the exam or re-submit the assignment. You need to be able to identify what it is that went wrong and address this. Often students do not address the problem and just hope that the examiners will be sympathetic to the re-submission. This is a dangerous strategy. Box 7:13 gives students a path of guidance on how to cope with setbacks.

## Box 7:13    Practical Help with Examination Setbacks

- Make an appointment to see your personal/academic tutor as soon as you receive your results.
- Your tutor will discuss your options with you, for example, re-sits or re-submission of assignments.

*(Continued)*

*(Continued)*

- If you feel your examination or assignment result was unfair, or you are unhappy with the advice from your personal tutor, you may take further advice from staff within the school/department. In addition to this you can discuss your concerns with the college/university student support department or the Students' Union.
- Some institutions have a 'progress' committee (it may be given a similar name). This is a representative group of academics from across the college/university who interview those students who have not been successful enough to progress to the next stage of their course. If you have been asked to attend such a committee you will be given details well in advance of what is expected from you. You may take a representative with you, and you are usually allowed to take a supportive friend. We understand the anxiety caused by such committees, but we ask students to be aware that the members are there to act in the interests of the student.
- We strongly advise you to make regular appointments to see your tutor for tutorials to help with preparation for exam re-sits and assignment re-submissions. Obtain as much feedback as you can from your work.
- Keep positive, address the problem and do not wallow in self-pity.

Unfortunately, a small number of students will fail an assignment or exam and when this happens it is a natural reaction to be angry and, perhaps, a little ashamed. The single most important thing to do is to get through this initial response and bring a more logical and objective analysis of what went wrong. Be mature, and ask yourself whether you revised enough, filled your 'reservoir' of knowledge enough and planned appropriately. Was your revision logical and systematic or were you haphazard and engaged in avoidance strategies? Could you have done any more? If this honest approach reveals the crux of the problem then it is important that you address this for the next time. If you feel that you had done sufficient and that you could honestly not have done more then the problem is likely to be exam technique and the management of anxiety. Talk to your personal tutor and ask advice, and re-read this book and practise the strategies that we have suggested.

## Had a Setback?

Get through your anger.
Identify what went wrong.
Address the problem.
Get positive and show them what you can do.

# Conclusions

We conclude this chapter by reasserting that there is no 'magic' in passing exams and assignments. Neither is there an 'x' factor to success in theoretical assessments. Passing exams and assignments is dependent upon a logical and thorough preparation in all of life's domains. It is about acquiring a thorough knowledge about the rules and regulations of assessments and working steadily over a period of time, building up a 'reservoir' of knowledge and confidence. If you have performed poorly in the past at exams, we suggest that you put those experiences behind you and start with a positive attitude – from today!

## SUMMARY POINTS OF CHAPTER 7

- Examinations remain an important method of theoretical assessment for students undertaking nursing studies.
- Preparation for examinations provides students with helpful tips to achieve their goals.
- Understanding the rules and regulations of examinations helps students prepare and become more confident.
- Students are often anxious as they struggle to find time to prepare and revise for their exams.
- Coping with disappointing results is a challenge which can be relieved by employing appropriate strategies.

# Test Your Study Skills ...

1. What are the rules and regulations of your institution regarding examinations? (see page 139)

2. What do you know about the rules regarding sickness, absence and failing examinations? (see pages 136 and 138)

3. What factors do you have to take into account when preparing for exams? (see pages 124–131)

4. How do you write a revision plan? (see pages 125–126)

5. What is the role of the invigilator? (see pages 139–140)

6. What are the roles of the first and second markers? (see pages 133–134)

7. What is the role of the external examiner? (see page 134)

# Practical Session ...

1. Inform your family/partner of your examination dates.

2. Enter the dates on your study diary/plan.

3. Organise a revision plan well in advance.

4. Organise additional care for those you have a special responsibility for.

5. Attend any exam technique seminars/lectures that are offered.

6. Arrange to see your personal tutor if you have any exam issues you wish to discuss.

7. Use the library facilities to increase your knowledge for both assignments and examinations.

8. You may feel you would like a practice exam; your tutor can arrange this for you and give you constructive feedback.

# 8 Theory and Practice

## LEARNING OUTCOMES

1.  To understand the relationship between theory and practice.
2.  To appreciate the potential for viewing theory and practice as one conjoint activity.
3.  To be able to analyse the constructs of an argument.
4.  To be able to construct a logical argument.
5.  To know how to produce ideas rooted in practice.

## Introduction

In many walks of life we often talk of the difference between theory and practice, and certainly at a simple level we are clear that there *is* a difference between them. We often hear phrases such as 'well, that's all right in theory …' and 'yes, but in practice …', which clearly indicates that we know what we mean by the terms theory and practice, and that there is a clear difference between them. In nursing we talk about the 'gap' between theory and practice in relation to the delivery of nursing care, which again not only suggests that they stand at opposite poles to each other but that the difference between them can be narrow or wide. However, it is not always clearly understood what exactly are the distinguishing features of theory and practice.

In this chapter we will examine the relationship between theory and practice by establishing the principle that all human action is underpinned by some degree of theory. The development of practice is dependent on ideas and concepts that are tested by research and we will examine these constructs of theory and reveal how they interlink. Part of the process of developing practice involves the role of argumentation and we will highlight how this is logically constructed. This will then be linked into both nursing theory and nursing practice.

# Theory and Practice: An Example

Let us think of an example of human action that incorporates theoretical components and practical behaviour. Imagine a primitive cave-dwelling group whose task for the day is to hunt and catch a wild animal to provide food for the small clan of cave people. Before they set out, they may perform a ritual dance, prayer or sacrifice to put the gods on their side and to increase their good fortune. The group perform this ritual because they believe that the gods can influence good or bad hunting and that the dance, prayer or sacrifice is related to pleasing or displeasing the gods. For us in modern times the behaviour may be viewed as 'superstitious' but for the cave people it would be considered to be sound reasoning. We may view their theory as flawed but they would hold it to be true. Now, if the hunters then went out and sought their prey by crouching and stalking, circling it to be downwind, setting traps, making noise to drive it towards the killers, etc., this too has both theoretical and practical components. The theoretical aspects involve being quiet during the stalking so as not to be heard or seen by the prey, to be downwind so that the wind does not carry the smell of the hunters to the prey, ensuring that the traps will hold or kill the prey, and so on. Thus, the practical action of catching the prey has a complex theory to it that has been developed over time, and the more understanding the hunters have of the theory of hunting the more chance they will have of catching the prey. This will lead to a better chance of survival and a more developed cave community. We can see that the cave hunters' 'theory' of hunting involves what we may consider partly unsound and partly sound theories, but that they would consider it, in its entirety, as totally sound.

## Learning Aid

Why do we believe in the latter theory of hunting (quiet, stalking) and not the former (praying to gods)? What are the differences between the theories?

Although we have used an example of a primitive cave group, there are people today who continue to hunt by these methods. Furthermore, the relationship between their theory and practice remains the same as it does in all human action, including human behaviour in healthcare settings, and more specifically as it does, for us, in the delivery of nursing care.

In the modern healthcare setting it is, perhaps, uncomfortable for us to consider that nursing action may be based on 'flawed' theoretical thinking. Indeed, we expend some considerable effort to ensure that nursing care is underpinned by sound scientific principles. Yet, we can note many differences of opinion between many nurses in relation to what nursing action is best in particular situations. For example, despite modern science there remain divided opinions regarding the most appropriate nursing action to heal pressure sores.

## Learning Aid

What aspects of nursing behaviour can you identify as not having sound theory underpinning it?

The important point to note is that nursing practice should, as all practice should, be based on sound theoretical principles.

# What do we Mean by Theoretical Constructs?

Theory is concerned with mental ideas, concepts and notions, which go to form an explanatory system about something in the external world. For our purposes the constructs of a theory are critical thinking, the synthesis of ideas and their utilisation. The first construct, critical thinking, itself has a number of sub-elements but broadly speaking refers to how we analyse a particular thing, statement or event by examining its arguments, relationships and logic. (Our caveman emerges from his dwelling and notes the wind is in the 'wrong' direction but the season of the year is 'right' for hunting, the temperature is within the range but the rain will make it difficult.) Many people say many things which often contradict each other, therefore we need mechanisms by which we can look beyond the superficiality of mere statements. Critical thinking assists us in this, and is concerned with not taking things at face value and understanding that there are usually, at least, two sides to every point of view. (Some members of the tribe say the 'gods' are with them, others say they are angry; some say the omens are bad, others that they are good; some say they should try a new hunting area that they have heard is good, others that they are starving and should hunt in traditional grounds.) We often read research papers that present a series of findings, followed by the drawing of conclusions. If we took every research paper at face value we would soon be totally confused as to the nature of the world. So, we need to be able to think critically about the research studies and examine if the parts are logically constructed, if they are related to each other in a sound manner, and if there is a link between, say, the findings and the conclusions that are drawn. However, to do this we need to know the structural components of the research process itself and have some knowledge of how they are related to each other.

## Learning Aid

Learn the constituent parts of the research process and understand how they are related to each other.

## Theoretical Constructs?

Ideas.
Concepts.
Theories.

## Arguments

In the academic world the term argument goes beyond the meaning that we normally assign to it when we use the word in our everyday world. In this latter application the word argument has negative connotations (as in being 'argumentative') and when viewed in this manner there is a question raised as to how sound the reasoning is of that argument. This now gives us a clue as to how we use the word argument in academic circles. In this environment it has a much more positive interpretation whereby the construction of an argument is viewed as an academic skill. However, in these circles, arguments are examined carefully for their reasoning, their logic and their soundness. In developing arguments we are attempting to *persuade* someone about something and we are engaged in constructing a theory about a practical action. Take a look at Box 8:1 and note that the speakers are clearly in disagreement with something, but also note that they are not constructing an argument based on reasoning, nor are they making an attempt to persuade us to our way of thinking.

## Box 8:1   Comments of Disagreement

'I don't agree with the new policy on taking annual leave. I think we should be allowed to take it when we want.'
'They say that people should have a balanced diet but I think that people should eat what they want.'
'That new way of bandaging is hopeless. I think we should go back to the old way.'

You are not likely to change your mind as a result of the above comments nor are you likely to alter your behaviour. They are statements, or points of view, but they are not arguments.

## Learning Aid

Why would you not be persuaded by the comments in Box 8:1? What would persuade you?

In building an argument we would have to include such phrases as 'because of …' or 'due to …' in our examples in Box 8:1 to provide a structure of reasoning. Box 8:2 shows how this might now look.

We can see from Box 8:2 that the speaker is beginning to develop their argument a little more, and whilst there is no attempt to make their point of view in a forceful manner there is an attempt at persuasion.

## Box 8:2   Reasoning Comments

'I don't agree with the new policy on taking annual leave, because it is too restrictive and doesn't allow people to plan ahead. I think we should be allowed to take it when we want as this will raise morale and give people a degree of control.'

## Learning Aid

Make a counter-argument against the reasoning in Box 8:2. You can use phrases such as 'since …', 'in spite of …', 'because …', 'due to …', 'given that …', 'seeing as …', 'in view of the fact that …' and 'while …'.

Arguments also need a conclusion, which is, in one sense, the main point that is being stressed.

## Learning Aid

Conclusions do not always come at the end of an argument; they can come at the beginning or in the middle.

Take another look at the comments in Box 8:2. The conclusion, that is the main point of the comment, is the second sentence. It is where the argument is going, it is the whole crux of the matter for the speaker. You can recognise an argument by trying to understand what it is that the speaker is attempting to establish. Arguments at one level or another are used in many areas of life from the playground to the courts and from the tabloid newspapers to the scientific journals. Even a bad argument is nonetheless an argument if it has the constructs of an argument (i.e. reasoning, conclusion and persuasion). In academic circles, as well as many other areas of life (e.g. politics), we use arguments and counter-arguments to express a point of view, and these are then measured for their logic and persuasion. In studying nursing, or any other subject, you will need to have the ability to construct arguments as well as to identify other arguments that are being put forward by others. Listening for arguments as well as constructing them is a skill that needs to be learnt. Therefore, the more you do it, the more skilled you will become. In writing an assignment (see Chapter 5) you will often be asked to construct arguments and counter-arguments. For example, when asked to 'discuss' or 'examine' a particular topic you are being tested as to your ability to balance the arguments and draw the logical conclusions from them.

In constructing arguments we need to be able to distinguish between argument, explanation and summary. Remember that an argument needs reasoning, a conclusion and persuasion. However, some arguments are not really arguments at all, despite having the appearance of being so. Box 8:3 shows a comment that has the appearance of being an argument, but actually it is not.

## Box 8:3    Explanatory Comments

'The surgery will open late at 1800 hours. This is due to sickness and there is only one receptionist available. The surgery will stay open later to clear any backlog of patients still waiting to be seen by the doctor.'

This does have the appearance of an argument as it has a conclusion and two reasons for it. However, it does not have any persuasive element to it, as it merely offers an explanation of what is going to happen. This is not to say that explanations are not useful in building theory; on the contrary, they are very important and are often required to support an argument. Read the comments in Box 8:4 and try to work out which statements are explanations, which is the conclusion, and what is the argument.

## Box 8:4    An Argument

'The surgery will open late at 1800 hours. This is due to sickness and there is only one receptionist available. The surgery will stay open later to clear any backlog of patients still waiting to be seen by the doctor. In an attempt to prevent this situation happening again we ought to have access to bank staff who can act as temporary receptionists. This will be cost-effective because we will be able to see more patients in a shorter time.'

Summarising is another way in which it may appear that an argument is being made but in fact this too lacks the persuasive element and therefore is not a true argument. Summaries usually have a series of points that can look like reasoning but the conclusion does not employ the points that are made as a reason for the conclusion and therefore is not an argument. Box 8:5 shows an example of this.

## Box 8:5    Summarising

'Choosing your course of study is an important decision in life. It will affect your future career and influence your perspective on the world. Furthermore, it is costly and involves a considerable amount of hard work. It will also affect your social life and determine your circle of friends. So, anyone making this decision will need to take their time and deliberate carefully.'

You can see here that the first four lines appear to be developing a line of reasoning as required in an argument but that the final sentence merely reiterates what has gone before, and does not attempt to persuade someone to a course of action. This makes the important point that we must understand the relationship between the reasons and the conclusion. The conclusion should be *drawn* from the reasons and the reasons should supply sufficient weight to support the conclusion. If they do not, then the conclusion is considered wrong or, at best, weak. What you are looking for in the relationship between reasoning and conclusion is the *relevance* of it. Box 8:6 shows a conclusion and some reasons for the statement.

We can see in Box 8:6 that all four reasons may in fact be true but that only reason (3) is strongly related to the conclusion. The other reasons would be considered weak.

> # Box 8:6    Relationship between Reasons and Conclusion
>
> **Conclusion** — There should be a clear health promotion policy against smoking tobacco.
>
> **Reasons** —
>
> 1. Many policies are confusing to people.
> 2. Health promotion is about 'policing' society.
> 3. There is a strong relationship between smoking and lung disease.
> 4. Some people smoke 60 a day for 60 years and do not suffer ill health.

Thus, in developing our theory of practice we need the ability and skill of argumentation and this not only involves building our own arguments but also incorporates the ability to examine other people's arguments.

## Building an Argument?

It needs reasoning, logic and soundness.
It needs persuasion.
It needs a conclusion.
It needs to be distinguished from explanations and summaries.

## Ideas

In building theory the notion of ideas is important and we take the word here to refer to concepts, theories, principles, laws, models, and so on. They are reflected in practice and can be generated by thinking about practice areas, what we do and asking why. Ideas have several interrelated sub-components: (a) making sense; (b) synthesising; and (c) utilisation. The first concerns taking in new ideas, which does not mean merely memorising something in rote fashion, but *making sense* of it. A mathematical equation would be a good example of this. We could simply learn the numbers and symbols and be able to repeat it accurately, but if we did not know what the relationship between the parts actually meant then it would not make sense to us. New ideas need to be explored and we should be constantly asking ourselves what something means in relation to something else. By this we mean that a certain nursing action will have a knock-on effect with other nursing actions and we need to be continually trying to think how one nursing action might be related to another.

## Learning Aid

When taking down notes in a lecture write down the main ideas that you think of whilst the lecturer is speaking, and after the lecture is over go over all the ideas and see how, or if, they are related to each other.

The second element is synthesising ideas. This is where you are thinking through the ideas and trying to create a scheme, process or structure. It is often the case that when thinking through a number of ideas we will synthesise something new or original from established traditional sources. We may start with a book or lecture and break it down into a number of main bullet points, and from this we may relate it to a number of other sources to create the synthesis. The third element is utilising ideas. By this we mean using ideas by putting them into practice and by discussing them with others. Although we can have inspirational moments when our mind suddenly has a 'eureka' idea which creates a great insight, it is more often the case that we have to work hard for these moments. They can be enhanced by utilising your ideas and changing nursing practice, testing them in the real world and possibly amending them as you proceed. Utilise them in an exploratory way with others: you may be surprised that others may offer a significant contribution to the development of your ideas. A good method for doing this is to use a flip-chart and have a brainstorming session with others. You can also employ sketches, road-maps, flowcharts and mind-maps; in fact, you can use anything that helps you in exploring your ideas.

## Having Ideas?

It needs to make sense.
It needs synthesis into a scheme, process or structure.
It needs utility by being put into practice.

# Nursing Theory

Numerous authors have mentioned the very important point that nursing theory cannot be considered in isolation but must be seen in a direct relation to practice. For example, Greaves (1984: 74) stated that 'in the development of a curriculum for nursing there is quite clearly a need for the relationship of theory to practice to be seen as equally important, interrelated and integrated into the very idea of nursing'. As more nurses engage in research there is likely to be an increase in the extent of nursing knowledge and more and more practice areas will be examined via scientific methods. Nursing action must be underpinned by clear thought, sound knowledge and clear, rational, theory. The idea of 'knowledgeable doers' is a term that resonates throughout nurse training, and comes closest to this principle.

## Hypothesising

We will finish this section by dealing with hypothesising. Although when taken in its literal scientific sense this refers to questioning the relationship between two events and inferring whether this represents a cause-and-effect association, we can employ it in a broader way for our purposes here. When nursing action is questioned we can ask what might happen if we do not do a particular action, or what might be the result if we do something else. Once we have thought this through and arrived at a reasonable suggestion, then we can say that we have a type of hypothesis.

### Learning Aid

What aspects of nursing would you question? Why? What would you like to stop or change? What are the likely consequences?

Once you are in this position you can begin to test out your hypotheses in practice and if the nursing action in question is a serious matter then this would need to be formalised through the appropriate channels and via the correct method (e.g. policy change, audit, research, etc.).

## Practice Context

Given that we accept the principle laid down in our example of the cave people above, then all practice, that is, planned human action, is underpinned by theory of one description or another. We have already noted that this theory can be false (i.e. superstitious), or it can be considered to have varying levels of strength. However, the starting point is that the human action does have a theory to it. Thus, nursing practice of any type is also underpinned by theory, and now it is merely a question of unravelling what that theory is. However, this latter quest is the challenge for all nurses working in clinical practice, research and education, and is not for us to deal with in this book.

What we need to do is to set out the relationship between the practice context and the theoretical constructs outlined above. It is this relationship between practice and its theory that is so important to the developing profession, and that must be the focus of constant and intense examination.

At this point we would like to emphasise the importance that is placed on clinical skills in nursing practice, and these are highly valued by both nurses and patients. Much clinical expertise is acquired through practical experience. We are aware that many nurses, particularly those returning to practice, feel that their years of nursing experience appear to count for very little in a profession which has changed and is now fundamentally both driven and led by research. We believe that many of the 'traditional' practices that have been passed down from one generation to the next continue to have a significant impact on the quality of care that nurses provide. The reality is that the nursing profession is enriched by a combination of practical experience based upon traditional nursing methods and a new evidence-based ethos.

All nursing practice is important and can be the pivot for developing theory. It is often the case that practices are reflected upon, as we will see in Chapter 10, and stimulate thoughts about their effectiveness or otherwise. This can then lead into establishing a theory concerning why this may be the case or what changes may need to be undertaken. Furthermore, whilst this ability to theorise from practice is important, we cannot undervalue practical knowledge itself.

## Learning to Theorise

For some, the answer to this sub-heading may be obvious but for others it may be less so. We often hear nurses complain that they do not know how to develop research ideas or cultivate topics for projects, and so on. Yet, the practice of nursing is replete with issues, practices, policies and procedures that have largely remained unexplored. One only needs to consider a day's (or night's) shift and think through all the events and actions that you undertake, and then ask yourself what theory is likely to underpin it.

## Learning Aid

What theory might underpin the nursing handover at the beginning/end of a shift?

With certain nursing action it may be clear what theory may support it. For example, taking a patient's temperature, pulse and respiration is clearly underpinned by the numerous theories related to an increase in temperature and infection or a reduction of temperature and hypothermia, pulse rates and the various conditions related to them, and the problems encountered with high and low respiration rates. These are long-established theories and have a clear relationship to why we undertake the observations. Applying dressings, splints and bandages are also nursing actions that have sound theories underlying them. However, much of nursing practice has an apparently amorphous and nebulous relationship to theory and is embroiled within a social or interpersonal perspective, which makes an examination much more difficult to undertake. Although we may accept this difficulty, this is not to say that it cannot be undertaken or that it should be avoided. On the contrary, it is imperative that all nursing action is scrutinised, and scrutinised effectively, according to scientific principles. If we take, as an example, the 'Learning Aid' question above relating to the nursing handover, you may have suggested that it is underpinned by theories relating to effective communication or sociological theories of organisational analysis. Or, you may have suggested that it is theoretically related to the psychology of team building, confidence boosting, raising morale and reducing stress. One or all may be correct but the important point is that the handover is a nursing action that does have underlying theoretical principles to it. In beginning to scrutinise nursing practice you need to be creative and constantly ask yourself why such and such an action is being done and what theory might explain it. Box 8:7 gives some hints and pointers as to where to look and learn to theorise.

---

## Box 8:7   Where to Look and Learn to Theorise

- During lectures.
- Watching a demonstration.
- Watching television/video.
- On the computer.
- Listening to the radio.
- Watching the news.
- In discussions with friends and colleagues.
- During a seminar.
- Having a brainstorming session.
- During a problem-solving exercise.
- Engaging in a role-play exercise.
- Interviewing someone.
- Reading a book or journal.
- Writing an assignment/project/case study.
- Engaging in debate.
- Reading lecture notes.
- And so on ...

## Learning to Theorise?

Scrutinise nursing action.
What theory underpins it?
Think about changing it.

# Doing and Theory

The importance of doing should now be obvious, from our cave people above to our nurses in the handover. The importance of practical action has been studied by many people for centuries, from the early Greek philosophers to the numerous scientists of contemporary times. This importance can be viewed on three levels. First, the science of doing is based on what is known as empiricism, which means gaining knowledge through experimenting, making observations and the acquisition of experience. Thus, practical action needs to be tested by scientific means, it needs to be scrutinised through meticulous observations and needs to develop through experience. You cannot do this unless you are trained in scientific methods. This is why research is important to nursing study.

Experience is only worthwhile if you do something with it; therefore, it needs to be ploughed back into action. This will enable nursing practice to develop alongside the other healthcare professions.

The second level of importance is concerned with responding to events in the real world. Remember that a model, or scientific theory, is only an approximation to the real world and that even with the laws of physics things do not always turn out quite as expected. Applying theories to practice is important so that we can test their application and gain the experience of their results. This helps us to respond to changing events as they occur. For example, when a cardiac arrest suddenly occurs, those with experience of dealing with this emergency can usually respond more appropriately than those who have none. The third level of importance concerning doing and theory involves the notion of actively making sense. When you engage in a practical action that you are unfamiliar with your mind is forced into thinking about its component parts. It will constantly be trying to work out how the action is to be achieved and how it can be done more effectively. This will continue until your mind is satisfied with the practical execution of the procedure. Once this state is achieved you can fall into the trap of 'doing something without thinking about it' or it becoming 'second nature' to you. Remember our example of driving a car without concentrating!

You need to develop the skill of looking at doing a particular action even when you are familiar with it, and you also need to broaden your experience by doing many different things related to your field of nursing and area of study.

## Learning Aid

Make a list of areas of experience in which you need to enhance your skills. These may include computer courses, presentation skills, public speaking, etc. Identify how you can achieve this improvement.

## Putting Ideas into Action?

Using science.
Responding to events.
Actively making sense.

# Nursing Process and Nursing Practice

The development of the Nursing Process can be seen as an attempt to apply a systematic analysis of nursing care to an individual's specific needs. Kratz (1979: 18) defined the Nursing Process as 'a problem solving approach to nursing, involving interaction with the patient, decision making and carrying out care based on the assessment of an individual patient's situation, followed by an evaluation of the effectiveness of our action'. We can see in this definition an interrelated mix of nursing actions, scientific evaluation, assessment of effectiveness, further influences on action, and so on. In short it highlights many of the issues that we have dealt with throughout this chapter. Greaves (1984) argued that it can be applied at three distinct levels. First, as a *simplistic application,* in which care of the patient can be planned at a standard level; second, as an *intermediary application,* in which care is planned in a more in-depth way; and finally as an *advanced application* in which theories of nursing can be used to plan care. Although the Nursing Process met with some resistance in the UK, and is no longer taught in many nursing departments and schools, it is worth pointing out its basic structure. The Nursing Process has four elements to it. The first is concerned with an assessment (A) of the needs of the individual, and the second with the planning (P) of care to meet those needs. The third aspect concerns the implementation (I) of that care and the fourth element involves an evaluation (E) of how effective it has been. Simply stated, this reflects a 'scientific' method of nursing care delivery and will probably resonate with those who are more familiar with problem-based learning approaches.

## Doing Nursing?

Assessing it.
Planning it.
Implementing it.
Evaluating it.

# From Classroom to Clinical Practice

The relationship between nursing theory and nursing practice has been studied in relation to how student nurses learn. Whilst formal nursing knowledge may be taught in the lecture theatre, the technical aspects are more likely to be taught in the clinical areas. This is not to say that the technical skills cannot be rehearsed in the classroom but merely that they will not be fully 'learnt' until they are applied in the real practice world. For example, we might learn to take a person's blood pressure in the classroom, but doing it in the clinical setting 'for real' will reveal added dimensions to it and various relations of importance to other procedures will be better understood.

# Conclusions

Many people view theory and practice as distinct elements, and indeed at one level they are. However, we have shown in this chapter that they can be viewed as one conjoint activity with each influencing the other. It has been argued that theory underpins practice and that all practice should be examined for theory. We have attempted to highlight strategies to enable nurses to engage in critical thinking about nursing practice and these have included constructing arguments and applying scientific methods. Finally, we have emphasised the importance of nursing practice as a source of investigation and suggested that the development of the nursing profession is dependent on how we evaluate our practice.

## SUMMARY POINTS OF CHAPTER 8

- The relationship between theory and practice is understood by the principle that all human action is underpinned by some degree of theory.
- The constructs of theory, when examined, reveal that ideas, concepts and theories are interlinked and interdependent.

*(Continued)*

*(Continued)*

- The logical construction of argument and its constituent parts is fundamental to understanding theory–practice.
- Understanding the connection of nursing theory with practice helps students relate their clinical experiences to academic work.

## Test Your Study Skills ...

1. What are the three main components to an argument? (see page 152)

2. What is the difference between arguments and explanations? (see page 150)

3. Why is a summary not an argument? (see page 151)

4. What are the three main sub-components of ideas? (see page 152)

5. Why is it important to examine nursing practice? (see pages 158–159)

6. What are the three levels of importance of practice (doing) and theory? (see page 157)

## Practical Session ...

In a clinical area ...

1. Identify a specific nursing action that you would like to change.

2. Write down the underpinning theory of it.

3. Establish what you would wish to replace it with.

4. Write down how you would test if your replacement action had been effective.

# Students with Special Needs

## Introduction

The term 'special needs' is intended to be a constructive one. In reality however, the experience of being labelled as a person with 'special needs' can be quite different. When our world is at its worst, it is completely unaware of and indifferent to people with special needs. By contrast, at its best, it can be all-embracing, where everyone works together, promoting the potential of each individual person. Most of the time, we manage something in between, where people with special needs are acknowledged but prevented from reaching anywhere near their full potential because of various shabby and inadequate yet essential mechanisms of support. It is little wonder then, that students with special needs considering moving into higher education may not do so because they imagine that student life may be even more difficult than it is in the rest of society. Pause for a moment and imagine you are a student who experienced a miserable time at school because your dyslexia was not recognised, understood or supported. You could be forgiven for thinking that university might be even less understanding of dyslexia and other special needs. If a student with special needs enters a nursing programme, anxious and with little expectation of support, it may be because they have already travelled a difficult journey with many unnecessary hurdles to overcome.

Many students will have had their special needs for a long time. They will have overcome significant challenges that their particular 'condition' brings. Other students may only realise that they have special needs such as dyscalcula (inability to deal with numbers) when they are university students. Therefore, special needs can be a fluid experience. For example, a student may have mental health problems in year two, but they may be resolved by the end of year three. There are different types of special needs, requiring varying degrees of support. Of course it also possible for students to have more than one special need – such as asthma and dyslexia – and this causes additional stress and requires support from various personnel in the university.

As we write this chapter we can report with some confidence that students with special needs are now regarded as integral to the wider community of higher education. In the last decade, institutes of higher education have travelled a long way and their knowledge of special needs has grown at the same time, offering increased support and expertise to all students.

The university population no longer consists of the tiny selected group of 18–25-year-olds at the apex of the educational pyramid. Students enter university at all stages of their life with varying qualifications and experiences. This chapter introduces special needs to nursing students and their lecturers, aiming to inform, discuss specific issues and provide further reading. It may be that finally we have a university population that reflects and embraces the diversities of the society in which we live.

# Access

Access for disabled students is covered by the Disability Discrimination Act (DDA) (1995). There is an obligation under this act for service providers to ensure adequate access for those with disabilities. It is unlawful for a service provider (a) to refuse to serve a person with disabilities for any reason relating to their disability; (b) to offer a sub-standard service to people with disabilities; and (c) to provide or offer a service on different terms. Service providers must make 'reasonable adjustments' so that persons with disabilities can use the services more easily. There are three broad types of 'reasonable adjustments': (i) changes to practices, policies and procedures; (ii) provision of 'auxilliary aids and services; and (iii) making the service accessible by another means. Access to buildings where services are provided must be made unproblematic by removing a physical feature, altering it to make access possible, or providing a means of avoiding a feature that makes access difficult.

# Disclosure of Disability and Confidentiality

Issues of disclosure and confidentiality tend to arise when the disability is not apparent and does not appear to affect the person's performance outwardly on a day-to-day basis. For example, if the person is physically disabled in some way and the impairment is overt for all to see, then disclosure and confidentiality are less likely to be an issue. However, if the disability is hidden from view and not obvious to others, then disclosure and confidentiality may feature large as issues of concern. Furthermore, it should be stated at the outset, and quite clearly, that if a disability is not disclosed then claims of discrimination under the Disability Discrimination Act (1995) cannot be made.

## Discriminating Against Disability?

According to the Disability Discrimination Act (1995), discrimination can occur by

- treating a person less favourably because of their disability, or by
- failing to make reasonable adjustments when a disabled person is placed at a substantial disadvantage.

To complicate matters it is incumbent upon a university to attempt to ascertain if a student has a disability in order that adjustments can be made so as not to treat the student less favourably.

## When the University Staff Should Find Out and Make Adjustments

When the student applies for a programme of study.
On application for accommodation.
At matriculation (enrolment at the college/university).
When placements, study trips, field notes are planned.
When undertaking a course requiring assessments/examinations.
When meeting the director of studies, programme leader, personal academic tutor.
When a student displays unusual behaviour.

In terms of disclosure, although there is a duty to find out if the student has a disability, they should not be asked unless there is a need to (DDA, 1995). This makes the 'waters' extremely muddy, but to assist those dealing with the issues the safer position is to tell only those people who need to know. Even not knowing does not exempt the university from responsibility as certain actions need to be taken in any event.

## Learning Aid

The university should…

Train staff in disability issues.

Provide guidelines to visiting lecturers, etc.

Make websites accessible.

Be prepared to provide notes and handouts in advance.

Ensure access needs are met.

Be prepared to provide information in alternative formats on request.

Look at each student as an individual.

Work with the student to ensure their learning needs are met.

Although it is incumbent on the university to find out if a student has a disability it may be that the student with disabilities requests that this information is kept confidential. Irrespective of this request, the university may need to make adjustments without informing others as to why these adjustments are made. It may be that the director of studies, personal academic tutor or student guidance and support may know of the disability but other academic staff and students are not informed. In the event of the disabled person requesting full confidentiality a number of steps may need to be taken.

## Possible Action in the Event of a Request for Full Confidentiality

The student is informed that there is no guarantee of full confidentiality.

Depending on the nature of the disclosure, a line manager may need to be informed.

The Disability Discrimination Act does not take precedence over the Data Protection Act or Health and Safety legislation.

In cases of genuine overriding issues of health and safety, and duty of care, then it may be appropriate to break confidentiality.

The university may be restricted in its ability to make adjustments that it could otherwise make with disclosure.

A written note should be taken of discussions between student and staff.

The written notes should be signed by both parties whenever possible.

# Rights

The notion of rights in our society features large at all levels, from the rights of the unborn child through to the rights of the dying. Furthermore, we embrace human rights, including the rights of prisoners, patients and staff, as well as animal rights both of pets and of farm animals. It should be stated from the outset that people with disabilities too have specific rights that they may or may not wish to exercise, but that they are also cradled within, and subject to, the remaining rights that exist throughout society. In this section we wish to out-line briefly three Acts of Parliament that influence the disabled person and refer the reader to several other areas of legislation that affect their rights.

## Disability Discrimination Act (1995)

The Disability Discrimination Act (DDA) (1995) defined disability as 'a physical or mental impairment which has a substantial and long-term adverse effect on the ability to carry out normal day-to-day activities (part 1, section 1–1). The question of the extent of disability is determined in part 1, section 2, which deals with disabilities that preceded the 1995 Act and the extent to which they may be considered permanent or long-term.

## Disability Discrimination Act (1995)

Part 1 – Disability – definitions.

Part 2 – Employment – discrimination by employers, enforcement,
   discrimination by other persons.

Part 3 – Discrimination in other areas.

Part 4 – Education.

Part 5 – Public transport.

Part 6 – National disabilities council.

Part 7 – Supplemental.

Part 8 – Miscellaneous.

With the developments of new acts there is usually a close interface with existing legis-lation and as the DDA (1995), part 4, deals with Education in relation to the person with disabilities it impacts on the Further and Higher Education Act (FHEA) (1992) and the Education Act (EA) (1994). The main impact is in relation to the adjustments that educational establishments need to make in response to the needs of people with disabilities. These adjustments may be physical, such as wider doorways, ramps, etc., or about provision, as in providing early handouts, different coloured paper, and so on.

## Data Protection Act (1998)

Data Protection Act (1998)

Part 1 – Preliminary.

Part 2 – Rights of data subjects and others.

Part 3 – Notification.

Part 4 – Exemptions.

Part 5 – Enforcement.

Part 6 – Miscellaneous and General.

This Act arose from the advancements in technology whereby vast amounts of personal information were being gathered and contained on computer databases. From medical records to business organisations and from employer files to banking institutions, the amount of data amassed is huge. Thus, the DPA seeks to establish principles and practices by which this data is stored and kept as confidential as required.

## Data can only lawfully be made public ...?

With the person's consent.

When deemed necessary under the DPA.

For court proceedings.

When concerned with rights and freedoms of others in the public interest.

## Special Educational Needs and Disability Act (2001)

The Special Educational Needs and Disability Act (SENDA) (2001) is divided into three parts and sub-divided into a number of sections.

## Special Educational Needs and Disability Act (2001)

Part 1 – Special Education Needs

    Mainstream education

    General duties of local education authorities

    Appeals

This Act establishes legal rights for students with disabilities at pre-16 and post-16 years of age in general, further and higher education provision. It is unlawful for educational bodies to treat those students with disabilities less favourably than those who are non-disabled, in relation to their disability (for example, someone with dyslexia not being given more time to sit an exam).

# Health and Safety Law

To ensure that wherever we work our health, safety and welfare are being protected we have health and safety legislation. It is the duty of the employer to ensure that the working environment is as safe as possible but it is also the responsibility of individuals to look after themselves and others at work. Thus, we can see that safe working involves a relationship between the individual, the employer and the law.

## Employers' Duties?

Ensuring a safe workplace without risks to health.

Making sure that workplace machinery and materials are transported, stored and used in a safe manner.

Ensuring that safe systems of operation are employed.

Making sure that you have information, instruction training and supervision.

Ensuring that you have adequate welfare facilities.

The employer is also responsible for carrying out risk assessments of workplaces and making reasonable adjustments where necessary. More specific responsibilities are also enshrined in law and include setting up emergency procedures, establishing first aid facilities, taking precautions against dangers, providing free protective clothing and equipment and reporting injuries, etc.

## Your Responsibilities?

Co-operate with employer.
Ensure that you take reasonable care.
Make sure that you use work items correctly.
Ensure that you do not interfere with or misuse items provided for your safety.

# Services

Universities, as well as other organisations, develop services not only for students and staff with special needs but also for all students and staff. Clearly, there are too many service developments to mention them all so we will briefly outline a small number here and advise the reader to check out the university that you are going to in order to establish the services that are available there.

**Personal Academic Tutor** – when you start at the university you may be allocated a personal academic tutor who will discuss matters with you relating to your academic development.

**Student Guidance and Support** – this service, in one form or another, is available at all universities and will have a wealth of information and contacts about all matters relating to students.

**Accommodation Services** – these may be available as separate entities or as part of a wider department (Student Guidance Support Services) and will have information relating to various types and availability of accommodation.

**Disability Equality Scheme** – The Disability Discrimination Act (2005) impose a statutory duty to promote equality for people with disabilities and universities are in the process of developing these schemes. Although these schemes may vary across universities, a number of developments appear to be emerging, such as networks of Diversity Advocates, Disability Link Tutors, Diversity and Equality Committees and Disabled Persons Sub-Committees.

**Finances** – a number of links have been established with various other university departments to provide information on finances including the Disabled Students Allowance (see Finances section below).

**Students Union** – this is another good source for many of the services for students both disabled and non-disabled.

# Finances

Disabled Students Allowances (DSAs) help with extra costs that you may incur because of your disability and as a direct result of your studying. Application can be made either before you start or during your course. The financial help that you receive does not depend on your income or on your family's income. Currently, help is available for the following:

Specialist equipment allowance up to £4,905 for the whole course.
Non-medical helper's allowance up to £12,420 each year.
General disabled students' allowance up to £1,640 each year.
Travel allowance to assist with extra travel costs.

# Nursing and Special Needs

In the relationship between educational establishments and disabled students there are a number of responsibilities.

The programme – Should not impede educational access.
      May be modified, e.g. notetakers, lab assistants, reduced course load.
      May change its instruction, e.g. brailled textbooks, handouts, extended exam time.
      Academic quality should NOT be compromised.

The tutor – Should not be unduly lenient.
      Should not grade more severely because of adjustments made.
      Should be fair and honest.
      Should be confidential.

The student – Is responsible for information regarding their disability.
      Should provide written medical evidence when required.
      Should be fair and honest.
      Should not abuse their disabled status.

# Points for Tutors

Acquire information on disabilities.
Ask the student with disabilities for their advice.

Make the course disability-friendly.
Acknowledge students with disabilities in course handbooks.
Plan to make appropriate adjustments.

Specific conditions may require specific adjustments and a few will be mentioned below.

## Chronic Illnesses

These may include asthma, diabetes, cardiopulmonary diseases, cancer, arthritis and neurological seizures. Under this heading we may also include chronic pain experienced in back/spinal problems, repetitive stress injury and post-surgical procedures. These may cause difficulties in walking, standing, sitting for long periods, limited energy and fatigue. The student may be on medication, which produces side-effects such as dizziness, confusion, lack of concentration and focus, dry mouth or blurred vision.

## Visual Disabilities

These vary considerably from needing glasses to complete blindness and from temporary disorders to permanent conditions. The problems may include reading textbooks, handouts, chalk boards, overheads, powerpoint presentations, watching demonstrations, and looking at computer screens and keyboards. The student may need large print, Braille, read-aloud facilities, note-taking facilities, talking calculators, preferential seating, modifications to presentations, and large-print handouts and presentations.

## Mobility Problems

These may include manual dexterity problems, multiple sclerosis, muscular dystrophy, spinal injuries, cerebral palsy and carpal tunnel syndrome. Students may need to use braces, crutches, walking-aids or wheelchairs. Students may be late for classes, need additional space, preferential seating, assistance in contributing in class (e.g. raising hand to gain attention) or changes in equipment, such as lower desks. We must remember that aids (crutches, wheelchairs) are essential to the person and should not be touched or moved without permission.

## Hearing Problems

These range from hardness of hearing to complete deafness and from a congenital condition to late onset. People with hearing problems vary in the ways that they communicate, including words, sign language, lip reading, facial expressions, known gestures and a combination of all these. Adjustments may include volunteers who type the spoken words on screen, various sound amplifiers and the traditional hearing aids. Tutors may wear micro-transmitters, speak facing the student and must remember not to speak when their back is turned to the deaf person. They should ensure that no more than one person at a time is speaking in group discussions. Students with hearing impairments may need preferential seating, advance notes or handouts, and volunteers to produce written notes.

## Dyslexia

Dyslexia is a disorder of reading and writing which is said to be brain-based rather than visual. The person affected usually reads at a significantly lower level than the non-dyslexic, despite having normal intelligence. The condition differs considerably from person to person and appears to vary in severity. There are usually difficulties with phonological processing, which involves the way in which sounds are managed, and therefore the person afflicted may have difficulty understanding what the tutor is saying. Adjustments are usually based on individual needs but revolve around educational tutoring. For example, it has been suggested that different coloured paper and inks affect the way that the dyslexic reads, so various coloured lenses can be attached to glasses and some corrective vision therapies have been recommended.

## Websites

Dyslexia – www..dfes.gov.uk/readwriteplus/understndingdyslexia/
Finance – www.direct.gov.uk/studentfinance
Chronic illness – http://illnesschronic.info/top.php?d=illnesschronic.info
Visual problems – www.prepare.org/disabilities/visualtips.htm
Mobility – www.tendringdc.gov.uk
Deafness – www.bbc.co.uk/health/conditions/deafness1.shtml

## Conclusions

Special needs is a term used to suggest inclusiveness rather than discrimination and various laws have been established to ensure fair practice in relation to student education. The main concerns are to ensure that students with special needs are not prejudiced against and for universities to make reasonable adjustments wherever necessary. These must be undertaken in conjuction with the student and in relation to the issues of disclosure of their disability and their right to confidentiality. University services have developed to assist students with special needs and is based on fairness, which is a two-way process involving universities making resonable adjustments and students with special needs making reasonable requests.

---

### SUMMARY POINTS OF CHAPTER 9

- Special needs is a term that is meant to be inclusive.
- Laws have been established to protect people with special needs.
- Students with special needs have a right not to disclose their disability but this may have repercussions.
- Students who do disclose their disability have a right of confidentiality within a framework of health and safety.
- Universities may need to make reasonable adjustments to assist students with special needs.
- University services continue to develop to assist students with special needs, which is based on fairness for all concerned.

## Test Your Study Skills ...

1. What are the three main Parliamentary Acts relating to Disability? (see page 165)

2. What is meant by Adjustments? (see pages 163 and 171–172)

3. When can data, under the Data Protection Act, be lawfully made public? (see page 166)

4. Name three services usually available for students with a disability? (see page 168)

5. What are the main responsibilities for students with a disability (see page 168)

## Practical Session ...

1. For students who are not disabled – attend your next class as if you were in a wheelchair and visit the toilet afterwards. How easy is access?

2. For students with disabilities – examine what practical measures could be taken to improve the student experience for you. Whom do you approach regarding this?

# 10  Reflection

## LEARNING OUTCOMES

1. To be aware of the variety of theories relating to reflection.
2. To understand the process by which reflection is undertaken.
3. To be able to employ the underlying skills of reflection.
4. To appreciate the role of both student and mentor in the reflective process.
5. To be able to write about the experience of reflection.
6. To understand the role of evaluation in developing change strategies.

## Introduction

Reflection has become a popular tool in nursing and it is now a learning requirement on numerous nursing courses, from basic training to post-graduate studies. However, in our experience some students dislike the exercises that accompany reflection and do not appreciate its relevance. One major reason for this is that students do not always know the underlying mechanisms of reflection and cannot relate its apparent theoretical process to any practical application. Furthermore, it is a central strategy in developing oneself in relation to clinical practice and by extension to the development of the profession. This chapter aims to provide the student with an appreciation of the importance of reflection by examining its central themes and, in particular, its relationship to nursing practice. Reflection is a systematic procedure that is logically constructed to provide a basis for changing practice, and is therefore considered to be a learning tool. Many organisms have the ability to learn, and this level of learning is a primitive one. It is often based on the stimulus–response model of learning as in Pavlov and his dogs, which learnt to salivate at the sound of a bell in the absence of the sight or smell of food. However, learning by reflection is said to be a higher-order level of learning that only humans possess. It is based on the ability of the human mind to 'bend back' on itself and think about thinking. It can take a particular moment in time and, in a sense, 'freeze it' in order to examine what one was thinking about at that time.

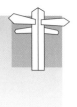

## Reflection?

A systematic procedure.
Thinking about thinking.
'Freezing' a thought.

In healthcare we are called upon to think about practices in a critical manner in order to ensure that we are providing a quality service. Reflecting on practice enables us to 'see' the constituent parts of a particular practice, and in this chapter we will outline both the theories of reflection and how the stages of reflection are developed. We will argue that reflection can be undertaken logically and analytically rather than by cursory thought. Reflection involves both the student and the mentor and we will explore this in relation to treating changes in practice.

## What Do we Mean by Reflection?

Our first task is to provide the reader with a definition of reflection from which we can build our discussion for the remainder of the chapter. There are a number of definitions and interpretations of reflection which we can draw upon to examine the concept.

## Defining Reflection?

A conscious process.
Interpreting from experience.
In isolation or with others.
Creates and clarifies meaning in terms of self.
Results in changed conceptual perspective.

We begin with the work of Boud, Keogh and Walker (1985), who have identified reflection as a process that is broken down into three stages. First, the experience is reframed and discussed with other people. Second, is the stage in which we work with others and deal with both positive and negative feelings, and the third, and final, stage is concerned with re-evaluating the experience and integrating new skills and knowledge (Boud et al., 1985). The development of reflection as a learning tool can be ascribed to John

Dewey, who is generally regarded as the founder of reflective thinking in relation to learning and education. Dewey defined the process of reflection as follows:

> Reflective thinking, in distinction from other operations to which we apply the name of thought, involves (1) a state of doubt, hesitation, perplexity, mental difficulty, in which thinking originates, and (2) an act of searching, hunting, inquiring, to find material that will resolve the doubt, settle and dispose of the perplexity. (Dewey, 1933: 12)

From these early days of developing the notion of reflection as a learning tool, we move on to the work of Donald Schon, who has made a considerable contribution to nurse education and practice through his writings on reflection (Schon, 1983; 1987). Crucial to Schon's ideas is the relationship between academic knowledge and professional practice. However, there are criticisms of Schon's work, particularly his narrow view of reflection and his lack of variety in the teaching situations that he described (Kember, 2001). We suggest that students spend some time reading Schon's work and have included his principal texts in the recommended further reading list (see p. 222).

## Models and Theories of Reflection

Models are usually produced developmentally with one person synthesizing the material of previous workers in the field and expanding on their concepts to create something new. The process is usually called progress. Some workers develop their own models over many years. Models of reflection are no different in this respect. Johns' (2000) Model for Structured Reflection is a good example of this. In this model the pivot is the shared experiences of both learner and supervisor, creating a greater understanding than reflection as a lone experience. Johns' model calls for the keeping of a structured diary, which should incorporate the following headings:

**Looking in** – thinking about your own thoughts and writing them down.
**Looking out** – analysing the situational factors and issues and writing them down.
**Questions – Personal, Ethical, Empirical**
   What were you attempting to do?
   Why did you respond as you did?
   What were the consequences?
   How were others feeling?
   How did you know this?
   Why did you feel the way that you did?
   Did you act for the best?
   What factors were influencing you?
   What knowledge informed you?

### Questions – Reflexivity

Does the situation have similarities with previous experiences?

How could you handle the situation differently?

What are the likely consequences of alternative actions?

Do you feel any different now about the situation?

Can you support yourself or others any better as a consequence?

Rolfe et al. (2001) outlined a Framework for Reflective Practice that employs Borton's (1970) Developmental Model. It is similar to Johns' (2000) model, in that it asks a series of questions under the three fundamental headings of 'What?', 'So what?' and 'What now?'

What …

is the problem?

is my role in the situation?

was I attempting to do?

action did I take?

was the response of others?

were the consequences for patient/self/others?

feelings were evoked in the patient/self/others?

was good or bad about the experience?

So what …

does this teach me for the patient/self/others?

was I thinking as I took action?

did I base my responses on?

should I have done to make it better?

is my new understanding?

are the broader issues?

What now …

do I need to do to improve things?

are the broader issues needing to be addressed?

are the consequences of my actions?

We now consider how we assimilate knowledge, and there are four basic ways that we understand how knowledge is constructed and employed in nursing practice.

## What is Reflection for?

Reflection is concerned with learning about something.

Learning is concerned with knowledge of something.

## Learning Aid

Can you reflect on something without learning about it?
Can you learn something without knowledge of it?
Can you know something without learning about it?

It would seem that the pivotal point is how we use the term knowledge (epistemology), and for our purposes here we can say that there are four basic ways that we understand how knowledge is constructed and employed in nursing. The first is empirical knowledge, which refers to knowledge that is derived from the external world from the application of scientific methods. It is considered to be natural, reliable and objective. An example of this would be knowledge gained through the research process. The second concerns interpretive knowledge, which is based on our understanding of lived experience in the world and it emerges from inside the person. It is knowledge that is considered to be subjective, experiential and not generalisable. An example of this would be a person's interpretation of a nursing action. The third is socially constructed knowledge that is based on the values and norms a given society holds. It is created through language, images and the symbols of our society, and is considered to be diffuse, interpersonal and contextual. An example would be the social construction of a teenage pregnant woman as immoral, sexually promiscuous and lacking in the values of our society. The fourth is critical knowledge, which is concerned with examining old ideas and practices in new ways and uncovering different levels of meaning. It is not too dissimilar to interpretive knowledge and socially constructed knowledge, and involves employing certain aspects of both these approaches. It is considered to be radical, emancipatory and empowering. An example would be feminist thinking that sees medicine as a male-dominated system.

## Learning Aid

There are many other types of knowledge and it is often the case that they overlap to some degree.

## Building Knowledge?

Empirical knowledge.
Interpretive knowledge.
Socially constructed knowledge.
Critical knowledge.

So, if types of knowledge can be said to exist, and knowledge is somehow dependent upon the philosophical perspective that the learner holds, then it can also be said to hold certain 'interests'. These 'interests' involve the personal perspectives of the individual and may be related to their belief systems, i.e. religious, political, scientific, etc.

## Learning Aid

Identify who the stakeholders are in a given encounter. Establish who has the power.

We are now in a position to consider some specific perspectives of reflection. In the context of professional education, reflection has a specific meaning as a complex and deliberate process of thinking about and interpreting experience in order to learn from it. This is a conscious process that does not occur automatically but is in response to experience of something with a defined process applied to it. Reflection can take place in isolation or it can be undertaken with others. Boud et al. (1985: 8) considered that 'reflection in the context of learning is a generic term for those intellectual and affective activities in which individuals engage to explore their experiences in order to lead to new understanding and appreciation'. Boyd and Fales (1983: 101) stated that 'reflective learning is the process of internally examining and exploring an issue of concern triggered by an experience, which creates and clarifies meaning in terms of self, and which results in a changed conceptual perspective'.

In an excellent book Taylor (2000) identified three types of reflection: (a) technical, (b) practical and (c) emancipatory. Technical reflection, Taylor argues, is based on empirical knowledge that is scientifically derived. It is considered to be logical, rational and based on deductive thinking about a particular nursing action. It involves rigorous scientific reasoning and application of scientific principles. Many nursing procedures can be examined in this way. Practical reflection employs interpretive and social knowledge, and is concerned with description and explanation of interactions. It often relies on the language and behaviour of people in an interaction and, again, many nursing activities can be examined via this method. Emancipatory reflection also uses the methods in practical reflection but is more interested in how people interpret themselves in social contexts. It focuses on the strategies by which people fulfil their roles and 'see' themselves functioning within them, and this may involve interpreting the relations of power by which they function. This type of reflection can be transformative, in that it can liberate a person from a particular role or behavioural restriction.

Another way of categorising reflective practices is that as outlined by Burns and Bulman (2000). These authors identify two main ways in which nursing knowledge can be elucidated. They suggested that reflection can be employed on, and in, action.

Reflection on action means thinking about something that has happened in the past, whilst reflection in action is concerned with how we recognise when something new to us is happening and we think about this whilst it is happening. We could add another category and that is reflection before action, which is concerned with thinking about something before it occurs, and might involve, say, the planning of patient care.

## Types of Reflection?

Technical.
Practical.
Emancipatory.
On action.
In action.

# The Roles of the Mentor and the Student

We begin this section by suggesting to students that reflection is a shared learning experience between students and their mentors. Historically, many qualified nurses did not benefit from mentorship during their training. Unfortunately, some students today also have only scant mentorship. We believe that such students had, and have, an impoverished learning experience as compared to those students who have the mentorship structure within their nursing programme. This section focuses on the individual and specific roles of first, the reflective mentor, second, the student and third, how these roles complement each other in reflective practice.

## Relationships in Reflection?

The reflective mentor.
The student.
In practice.

## The Reflective Mentor

For those involved in nurse education, defining what a mentor is continues to cause considerable debate, and many definitions have been put forward to try and resolve this dispute. We offer the definition of the English National Board (now incorporated by the Nursing and Midwifery Council) as a starting point for students and mentors to develop their own discussion: 'an appropriately qualified and experienced first level nurse/midwife/health visitor who, by example and facilitation, guides, assists and supports the practitioner in learning new skills, adopting new behaviours and acquiring new attitudes' (English National Board, 1990).

We appreciate that many qualified nurses will find reflective mentorship a daunting prospect. This is because 'reflection' is a relatively new concept in nurse education and many qualified nurses practising today were not taught reflective practice in their training. Today, however, as we say above, reflection is a fundamental learning tool embraced by nursing programmes at many levels of study. Students are required to fully engage in reflective practice within the clinical environment and demonstrate their ability to transfer this to the written word in theoretical assessments. To address this 'learning gap', those qualified nurses preparing to become mentors are taught reflective practice on their study days. New mentors will frequently assert that they have always learnt from their experiences and practised reflective mentorship, even though they didn't know it was called that! It is from this point of making the connection between believing that they always undertook reflection that qualified nurses begin to develop, and fine-tune, their skills of mentorship through learning that it is an active and deliberate process.

## Learning Aid

Reflective mentors can plan ahead for their students by creating
a learning clinical environment and developing their own skills in reflective practice.

Once nurses decide that they would like to become effective reflective mentors who can make a positive contribution to their students' learning experience, we suggest that they engage with a number of practical activities; these are identified in Box 10:1.

## Box 10:1   Practical Guidance for Becoming an Effective Reflective Mentor

- Keep a diary of reflective practice.
- Include your own clinical practice learning experiences.

*(Continued)*

- Also include your learning experiences and the learning experiences of your student within your role as reflective practitioner.
- Arrange formal and informal discussion groups and seminars with colleagues to exchange ideas and provide mutual support to fellow reflective mentors.
- Attend study days on reflective practice.
- Continue to read and develop your knowledge, through attending conferences and reading journals and books.
- Keep abreast of new research and ideas on reflection through reading the literature and engaging in discussion.
- Take note of students' feedback sheets from clinical placements.
- If you are having any difficulties being a reflective mentor for a particular student, discuss these difficulties with the student's personal/academic tutor who will be happy to offer additional support where necessary.
- Work towards developing a learning culture within the workplace.

One of the key roles of the mentor is to be able to create and facilitate reflective practice opportunities. Daloz (1986) has identified three main areas of work for reflective practitioners: first, to be supportive, second, to be challenging and third, to provide vision. We have used these key roles as a suggested framework of activity for reflective mentors and this is outlined in Box 10:2.

## Box 10:2    A Framework for the Activities of Reflective Mentors

- **Be Supportive** — Take time to get to know your student's individual strengths and weaknesses. Take time to listen to your student and give feedback. Provide learning opportunities within the clinical environment. Be able to support your student in an open manner. By making time to be with your student you have demonstrated that they are important and worthy of your individual attention. Give something of yourself.
- **Be Challenging** — By understanding your student's abilities, you can challenge their skills and knowledge base without threatening their confidence.
- **Provide Vision** — This may sound frightening to some mentors! However, all mentors can provide vision, through their ideas, thinking, activities and ambitions for themselves and others.

## Learning Aid

Challenging students in areas that they are not familiar with can undermine their confidence and can lead to anxiety and hostility. Get to know your students!

## The Role of the Student

To some degree we are all students of reflection and reflective practice. Today, in nurse education, the teaching of reflective practice is one of the learning tools which crosses all programmes. Students and lecturers continually learn and develop their reflective skills for both teaching and learning purposes. For many students their introduction to the theories and practice of reflection is usually at the beginning of their nursing programme and this is re-emphasised throughout the subsequent modules. Box 10:3 identifies the specific activities of the student of reflective practice.

## Box 10:3   The Activities of the Student in Reflective Practice

- Develop self-awareness by taking time to consider and understand your own thoughts and actions.
- Reflect on critical incidents and events on a regular basis, so that reflection becomes integral to your thinking.
- Practise new clinical skills and apply models of reflection to develop your learning experience.
- Spend time with your reflective mentor to work towards learning being a joint venture.
- Gain new knowledge of reflective practice through reading, attending seminars and conferences.
- Learn from feedback from reflective supervisors.
- Address particular challenges which may arise through discussions and tutorials.
- Discuss informally the experiences of reflective practice with fellow students.

## Learning Aid

Keep a 'reflective practice' file with details of papers, book chapters and course work; this will be invaluable for assignments.

## Don't Want To Do It?

Avoidance strategy.
Find it uncomfortable.
Feels awkward.

## Shared and Individual Learning experiences between Students and Reflective Mentors

The relationship between students and their reflective mentors can, in the early days, be a testing time. We appreciate that both parties, particularly if they are new to their roles, can be a little wary of each other. This often arises when they are relating to an experience where they could have acted differently. They select a personal experience, relate the story to others and think 'I wish I hadn't told them that!', by which time it is too late and the perceived damage has been done. By contrast, some people are very private by nature and prefer to reveal very little of their inner thoughts. The answer to this common problem of reflective practice is to say only what you feel comfortable with saying.

## Revealing Thoughts?

Think before telling.
Say only what you are comfortable with.
Set out rules of trust.
Establish confidentiality.

## Learning Aid

Do I feel comfortable in divulging this event in my life to demonstrate my understanding of reflective practice?

Illustration 10:1 demonstrates the individual and shared learning between the student and the reflective mentor.

## Process and Skills of Reflection

Learning takes place irrespective of whether or not we fully understand how it actually occurs. However, active learning, it should be emphasised, refers to the fact that it occurs more effectively when our attention is focused on what it is that needs to be learnt. This sounds so obvious as to be almost meaningless, and yet it is the central point of learning and, in this respect, the central point of reflection. Therefore, to reflect we must bring something under our attention, and if we do this as an act that is motivated by ourselves rather than a 'teacher' attempting to catch our interest, then it is likely to be more effective.

## Learning Aid

Think of an issue or event that you were involved in yesterday. This can be as simple as greeting an acquaintance. Hold the image in your mind and 'freeze' it. Replay it in your mind.

The process of reflection can be viewed as having a number of stages. The first stage is to focus attention on something. This can be an event, situation, encounter, and so on, which has left you feeling a little uncomfortable, upset, disturbed or perplexed. It may be a major event such as your role in dealing with a cardiac arrest, or a brief encounter such as an interaction with an impolite colleague. It may be concerned with moving to another clinical area or the difficulty felt at undertaking a new procedure. The important point is that your attention is drawn to it. The second stage of the reflective process is the awareness of feelings, which often emerges from the negative feelings and thoughts that we experience in a situation. When describing the situation it is important to include these thoughts, feelings, salient events and key features. The third stage involves a critical analysis of the situation, which is constructive and includes an examination of both feelings and knowledge of how the situation has affected the individual and how the individual has affected the situation. It is crucially important to focus upon positive feelings, as well as dealing effectively with negative feelings that may impinge on a rational consideration of the situation. The fourth stage is the development of a new perspective on the situation, which is a consequence of the learning process. This may result in the development of new attitudes or values, or a new way of thinking about something. The fifth stage is action, or a commitment to action, resulting from the learning process. Box 10:4 highlights the main aspects or stages of the reflective process.

> # Box 10:4   Main Stages of the Reflective Process
>
> - **Focus of attention** – Active process of bringing an event/situation under attention.
> - **Awareness of feelings** – Emergence of uncomfortable feelings and thoughts.
> - **Analysis of situation** – Stakeholders' interests, balance both positive and negative points of view, who gets what and why, examine power relations.
> - **Interpretation** – Creation of options.
> - **Innovation** – New interpretations, conclusions, attitudes, values.
> - **Action** – Commitment to change something.

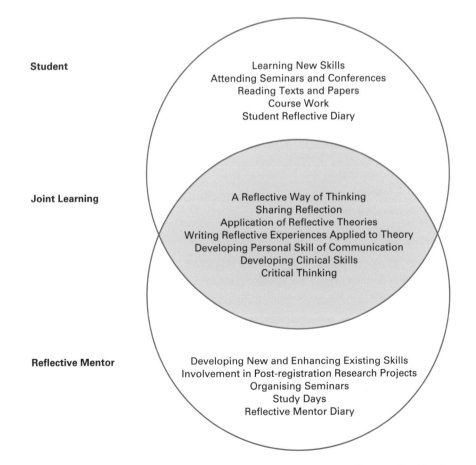

**Student**

Learning New Skills
Attending Seminars and Conferences
Reading Texts and Papers
Course Work
Student Reflective Diary

**Joint Learning**

A Reflective Way of Thinking
Sharing Reflection
Application of Reflective Theories
Writing Reflective Experiences Applied to Theory
Developing Personal Skill of Communication
Developing Clinical Skills
Critical Thinking

**Reflective Mentor**

Developing New and Enhancing Existing Skills
Involvement in Post-registration Research Projects
Organising Seminars
Study Days
Reflective Mentor Diary

**Illustration 10:1   Individual and shared learning between student and reflective mentor**

## Stages of Reflection?

What it is that you are thinking about.
What it is that you feel about it.
What are the components of it?
What else could be happening?
What are you going to do about it?

The underlying skills of reflective practice are similar to those required by the critical thinker, the student and the academic. They must be developed within the person, and the teacher of them can only provide examples and prompts. Many writers on the issue of the underlying skills of reflection tend to produce a list of general terms referring to the management of thinking. These may include attending to feelings and attitudes, developing self-awareness, using positive feelings, dealing with negative feelings, and so on. However, what these actually mean is often left to the imagination.

## Skills of Reflection?

Attending to feelings and attitudes.
Developing self-awareness.
Using positive feelings.
Dealing with negative feelings.

A better way of appreciating the skills of reflective practice is to use Burns' and Bulman's (2000) framework. This involves a five-element scheme for reflection in which the first is self-awareness. Self-awareness is important for many walks of life and it is vital in nursing. To be self-aware involves examining one's own feelings and identifying both negative and positive attitudes, thoughts and beliefs. It is also about seeing oneself in relation to how others 'see' you. The second element is description, which is the skill of accurate recollection of the important aspects of a particular event. It will involve the context, the sequence of events, the feelings and the outcome of the situation. The third element is analysis, which should be a critical engagement with the factors of a particular situation and the posing of a series questions about them. These may be: what happened; why it happened; who was involved; when it occurred; and so on. The fourth is synthesis, which refers to taking individual elements and building up something whole with them. It may involve a degree of creativity and original thinking.

## Learning Aid

Synthesis is not always an easy thing to do. A good tip is to try and make alternative interpretations.

The final element is evaluation, which is about looking back and making judgements. It often entails making a judgement about a particular value of an action or event. Box 10:5 highlights these main elements.

## Box 10:5    Scheme for Reflection (adapted from Burns and Bulman, 2000)

- **Self-awareness** – Examination of one's own values and how others 'see' you.
- **Description** – Accurate description of an event.
- **Analysis** – Critical examination of factors relating to an event.
- **Synthesis** – New interpretations.
- **Evaluation** – Making judgements.

Each of these elements can be seen to have sub-skills in the process of thinking, and although we may do them in our everyday world without really thinking about them they can be focused upon and developed as a skilled practice. In this way we sharpen our ability to think critically and this, in turn, helps us to develop nursing practice.

# Learning from Reflection

We have all, probably, had the experience of witnessing something that we have later felt was wrong and wished we had done something about it at the time. Furthermore, we have all, probably, had the experience of not inwardly agreeing with something but in the face of peer group pressure have kept quiet. In these situations we are measuring an action against our inner standards, values, norms and morals, and drawing a conclusion that something is good or bad, right or wrong, or not very good and could be improved. From this position of an inner assessment we then make an evaluation about how others would react if our inner views were made known. If we think that other people's reaction is likely to be negative then, depending upon the strength of our conviction and the importance that we consider the event to have, we are more or less likely to reveal our inner thoughts.

## Learning Aid

What minor action have you witnessed recently that you disagreed with but did not say, or do, anything about? This could be young children vandalising something or a friend or colleague saying something. Why did you not challenge them?

The assessment of response from others, of course, is complex and will incorporate such factors as the likely harm that may be received, which could be physical harm to self or psychological damage, or it could be damage to career, to family or to friends, and so on. Factors will also include the response of your conscience and how you are likely to cope with this. This is a very natural state of affairs in the human condition and should be understood, rather than dismissed or simply criticised.

## Learning Something from Reflection?

Keeping quiet when we should speak out.
Applying our inner standards.
Applying professional standards.

Reflective learning is a useful method of applying a logical approach to understanding human action, both small-scale and large-scale, and if employed correctly will make progress possible. The important point here is to engage in the method of reflection as a systematic process. Remember that the human mind will subconsciously work to protect itself against a guilty conscience by denial, repression, rationalisation, and so on, so reflection should be undertaken by shelving preconceived views. Reflection is not a cursory, nor quick, consideration of something, followed by a quick dismissal or denial, but a careful and considered mapping of an event followed by the logical drawing of conclusions.

## Defending our Egos?

Having a logical approach to understanding human action.
Assessing the mental defence mechanisms.

## Learning Aid

Assess a situation as a judge would. Take the evidence, weigh it carefully
and make a summary before announcing your decision. Give your verdict.

The major point to this section is that pure learning is not sufficient in itself; it must be accompanied by *action*, or at least a commitment to action. The commitment must be to create change, no matter how small and to do something different. By changing, by altering, by affecting, by influencing, we will make something better. This might be changing one's self in some way, changing the way that we behave to someone, or it may be changing the way that we do something. Once this has been undertaken we can then evaluate whether the change has made things better or worse. In short, we need to evaluate it. Learning from reflection also involves sitting down and writing notes, just as judges do.

## Learning Aid

The change strategy may fail. Do not be disheartened. Undertake reflection to
establish why. Have another go.

Evaluation is a vital part of the reflective process and should be undertaken carefully and honestly. It may be the case that the change that you have created has not had the desired effect or that the result is something that was not anticipated. If the change is evaluated as negative it is important that you do not become disheartened but see this as one cycle in the overall change strategy. Illustration 10:2 shows the cyclical nature of change and the role of reflection in it.

The evaluation strategy may incorporate a personal self-analysis as mentioned above but may also involve the use of others. Friends, colleagues, peers, patients and managers may all be asked to review whether a particular action is better or worse. You may also

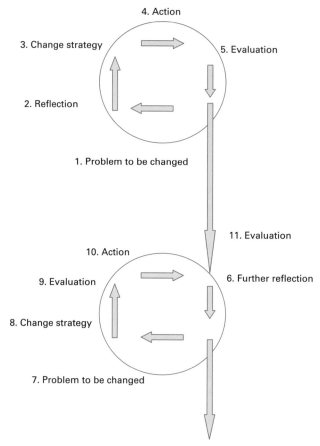

4. Action

3. Change strategy

5. Evaluation

2. Reflection

1. Problem to be changed

11. Evaluation

10. Action

9. Evaluation

6. Further reflection

8. Change strategy

7. Problem to be changed

12. Further problem to be changed

**Illustration 10:2  Cycles of change strategy**

wish to gather information regarding facts and figures relating to the change in practice as there may be records kept or reports made regarding this. Do not become defensive and try to remain positive.

## Changing Practice?

Action.
Commitment to action.
Evaluation.

# Thinking and Writing Reflection

We have seen throughout this chapter that the experience of reflection is an activity that weaves its way through our thoughts and thinking. We develop this process until it becomes part of us and contributes to our character and the kind of people that we are. It is customary for students to begin their reflective journey by talking about experiences and critical incidents that have had some impact upon them. Once students feel at ease with talking reflection and indeed listening about the reflective experiences of their colleagues, they can combine this with acquired knowledge of reflective theory and begin to write. In our experience, there are always a number of students who submit work that is little more than the recalling of an event. Writing is an active process and it is important to plan this carefully as we formulate our thoughts about reflection, but as Box 10:6 demonstrates, it is only a part of the overall process and should be undertaken as outlined in Chapter 5 on writing assignments. Furthermore, students who do submit purely experiential writing must expect to lose marks, especially if the assignment specifically asks for reflective theory. Thinking and writing reflection for academic work must be supported by the theories of reflection.

## Box 10:6    The Seven Stages to Writing Reflection

- **Stage 1** – Thinking about critical incidents and experiences.

- **Stage 2** – Sharing your thoughts with colleagues and friends.

- **Stage 3** – Developing your theoretical knowledge of reflection.

- **Stage 4** – Applying theoretical knowledge to your experiences and sharing these activities with colleagues and friends.

- **Stage 5** – Beginning to write a reflective journal.

- **Stage 6** – Practising reflective writing with different reflective models and incidents.

- **Stage 7** – Arranging a tutorial with your tutor to receive feedback from your reflective writing in preparation for your assignment.

To overcome the concerns frequently caused by writing reflection we suggest that students begin by keeping a reflective diary. We appreciate that the majority of students probably do not keep reflective diaries and the first time they write a reflective piece is for a module assignment. However, we strongly recommend that they do make an effort and diarise their experiences.

## Learning Aid

Practise reflective writing and get feedback from your tutor; this will help prepare you for your assignments.

Many programmes of study assess students' ability to write about reflection, particularly at diploma and undergraduate levels. The reflection may be within a specific module assignment such as psychology or it may be as part of a 'record of development', which many courses use to assess students' progress throughout their clinical placements. Nurses undertaking the return-to-practice course are also required to write a reflective piece on a critical incident that they have experienced on clinical placements. Box 10:6 gives students a phased approach to reach the stages of reflection from thinking to writing reflective practice.

Whilst we have suggested that students keep a reflective diary, we do appreciate that some people may be unsure as to how to begin this, or may even be embarrassed by the idea. Let us reassure you that the diary is for yourself, and your eyes only if you wish it to be. As a learning tool reflective diaries – or reflective journals, as they are sometimes called – have a number of uses. First, they form the basis of discussion with fellow students, tutors and mentors. We often find that the process of writing helps us to clarify our thoughts and you may find solutions to problems through this activity. You may also wish to compare your conclusions about an experience with other colleagues. Second, reflective diaries help students identify their academic needs; for example, they may need particular help with a subject or area of clinical practice that is difficult to them. Third, practising writing is a fundamental activity of any student (or lecturer!) and writing a reflective journal helps to develop writing skills. In Box 10:7 there are suggestions as to what students might include in their reflective diaries.

## Box 10:7    Suggested Ideas for Inclusion in your Reflective Diary

- Because a reflective diary is for you, you may write what you choose. It is the ideal place to write about your feelings, about your learning experiences, lectures, lecturers, fellow students, personal progress and ambitions.
- New challenges: for example, modules or clinical placements.
- New mentors or tutors.
- Changes in your home situation.
- New ideas that you may have about the course.
- Situations in which you learn the most.
- Situations in which you learn the least.
- Situations in which you can clearly link theory to practice.
- Worries, hopes and ambitions.

## Use of Reflective Diary?

Forms a basis of discussion.
Identifies academic needs in relation to clinical practice.
Develops writing skills.

When students begin their reflective writing, they are often unsure how to start. We suggest that students begin by reading Chapter 5, which covers in detail every stage of writing an assignment.

## Learning Aid

Are you maintaining your academic rigour in your reflective writing?

The structure of reflective writing is the same as for any other piece but there are some additional points for students to know when engaging in reflective writing; these are included in Box 10:8.

---

## Box 10:8   Writing Reflection: Points to Remember

- Follow the general rules of writing an assignment as discussed in Chapter 5. You are expected to write within a structure, including an introduction, a main body and a conclusion.
- Students will be used to being encouraged to write in the third person for their academic work. In reflective writing, however, the first person is the preferred form of writing. Practise writing in the first person and ask for feedback from your tutor. Avoid slipping into 'pub conversation', where your writing reads like a 'chat' rather than an academic piece of writing.
- Express your feelings about your experiences in a clear and well-thought-out way.
- Practise writing your analysis of your experiences in an articulate manner.

---

## Learning Aid

Don't attempt to write in the third person in reflective writing. Write in the first person but within an academic structure.

---

## Can't get Started?

Talk about experiences.
Write down feelings in private.
Keep a reflective diary.

---

Fortunately, there is a considerable amount of significant work that has been published on all aspects of reflection. We suggest that students make every effort to refer to some of these texts and papers, as some of them give examples of reflective writing, which will be useful in developing reflective writing techniques. The suggested reading list at the back of this book includes Benner, Boud, Rolfe and Schon, all of whom are significant workers in the field of reflection.

# Conclusions

Reflection is more than a casual thinking about something; it is a systematic process of analysing an action, event or situation. Learning to engage reflection in a logical way will enable the practitioner to identify actions and behaviour that require changing in one way or another. Through the process of reflection a change strategy can be devised, which will improve practice and thus, in turn, patient care. We have emphasised the point that reflection involves creating something new and innovative, and should be undertaken honestly and openly. Many find the process uncomfortable and become defensive about it. However, if done correctly it can be extremely helpful in professional development and can contribute significantly to changing practice.

## SUMMARY POINTS OF CHAPTER 10

- Reflection is a learning tool that can help us develop our theory and clinical practice.
- There are a number of theories of reflection, which students can employ to understand their clinical practice in a logical and analytical way.
- The roles of both the student and the mentor need to be understood for reflection to be an effective learning tool in the clinical environment.
- Students are required to be able to communicate their experiences of reflection through their writing, particularly in assignments.

# Test Your Study Skills ...

1. Name three types of reflection (see page 179).

2. Name the stages of the reflective process (see pages 184–186).

3. What is the role of learning in the reflective process? (see pages 179 and 181)

4. What is the role of the mentor in the reflective process? (see pages 179, 180 and 181)

5. What is the role of evaluation in the development of a change strategy? (see page 189)

## Practical Session ...

Identify a small piece of nursing action and ...

1. Go through the stages of reflection regarding it.

2. Write down notes on each stage.

3. Formulate a change strategy.

# 11 Personal and Professional Development

## Introduction

Studying incorporates many things and is not only about obtaining a particular quali-fication, although it is fair to say that most people predominantly study when under-taking a course of one description or another. Studying should be seen in a similar vein as, say, undertaking physical exercise. There are some who train to become Olympians and set their targets for a medal, and this, of course, means long lonely hours of intense effort and a rigorous change in lifestyle. Similarly, studying for a PhD can feel like this. However, most people who undertake physical exercise do so, not in the quest for a gold medal but merely because they wish to stay healthy. The enjoyment of physical exercise is not always felt directly before it is undertaken, nor is it felt during the ses-sion, but once completed it usually leaves most people feeling good and very satisfied. Studying can be viewed like this. It should be undertaken as mental exercise to keep your mind healthy, and should be balanced alongside physical work. You may not enjoy the prospect of it, nor find it easy whilst doing it, but the benefits will be felt once it is completed. Like physical exercise might be geared towards training for particular matches or events, and the overall season contributes towards a state of physical health, studying may be geared towards a number of courses or qualifications but taken over-all it is contributing to maintaining your mental health. In this chapter we will examine the reasons for engaging in study and analyse the relationship between clinical practice and professional development. Studying contributes to both personal and professional development and there are numerous benefits, which we will highlight. Lifelong learning is a common thread to modern healthcare delivery and we will discuss the importance of examining and developing your own career. Studying can form the basis of advancement and we will briefly outline some of the opportunities in nursing which can be explored with career ladders (see p. 209).

## Thinking about Studying?

Study for a course.
Study for health.
Study for professional development.
Study for the profession.

# Reasons for Study

There are many reasons for studying, but before we launch into these it is worth taking a moment to consider what we mean by the term study. Domerque (cited in Parnes, Noller and Biondi, 1977: 52) argued that 'some people study all their life and at their death they have learned everything except how to think'. This would indicate that there may well be a relationship between study and thinking but it is important to understand that this is not always necessarily the case. The suggestion is that learning to think is a skill in itself and study may assist us in learning how to do this. Therefore, we need to study to learn how to think and not just study to learn a mass of facts. We need to study in order to develop both ourselves and our profession, thus contributing to society in general.

## Learning Aid

There are many good books on learning how to think critically. Obtain one and read it carefully.

It is often the case that personal and professional reasons for studying overlap, or are even one and the same thing, but we draw the distinction between them as they can be seen as being separate motivations.

## Learning Aid

What motivates you to study? Is it distinctly personal or professionally motivated, or is it a mixture of both? Try to identify a weighting (e.g. 50 per cent personal, 50 per cent professional).

Now let us look at both personal and professional reasons for undertaking a course of study.

## Why Study?

Not merely to amass facts.
More important to study to think.

## Personal

There are as many reasons for studying as there are people who undertake it and it would be a pointless exercise to provide an extensive list of personal reasons. What we will do instead is to discuss some general rationales for study and examine some of the relations that often tie them together. One common personal reason for study that we often hear concerns intellectual development. Many people, particularly mature adults, may feel that they did not benefit from, or did not do justice to, their childhood education, and later in life feel that they would like to realise their potential. They may feel that they do not have enough knowledge, and yet feel inwardly that they have the potential to learn. Or, they may feel that they were somehow prevented from learning and would now like to address this. In these types of scenarios there is a gap between what they know and what they would like to know. This creates a tension, as they feel that they are in a state of ignorance and may feel embarrassed about this, or even anxious about it. This tension is related to confidence, in that they may feel anxious and apprehensive about their ability to undertake a course of study or pass an exam. However, frustrated intellectuals are usually highly motivated and enthusiastic learners, once they have overcome their fear of failure.

## Learning Aid

Identify what factors most concern you about studying. Write these down.
Identify which ones are personal issues and which ones practical issues. Write down a number of options for dealing with each one. Be proactive.
Putting it off will not solve it, nor satisfy you. You are important.

A second set of common reasons for studying may be bound up with what we may call career advancement. This may be based on a personal motivation to climb the ladder, which is a challenge to you, and reach higher positions in your profession. Of course, this is a laudable enterprise and many people feel this drive to get on. However, it may be that some people feel a necessity for study which is not due to a singular inner drive, but because of competition from others. In most professions there are many people chasing a relatively few positions and the higher up the profession one goes the more sparse the opportunities become (there can only be one chief executive, medical director, matron, etc.) in any one organisation. In modern times there is an emphasis on a balance between qualifications and experience, and not just on experience alone, which might have carried the day 20 years ago. This means that a greater number of people have more and more qualifications than ever before. This leads to a highly competitive marketplace and the motivation for study may well be grounded in the need to compete with others. Again, this is a laudable reason for studying and, whether you are a young student at the start of your career or a mature adult who is considering returning to study, you will certainly need further qualifications if you wish to compete for jobs in the modern healthcare setting. Finally, part of your motivation for study might involve the employer requiring you to do so as part of a legal requirement, or it may be that the line manager feels that you need a specific qualification in order to do the job. It may be that you have entered, or wish to enter, a specialised area of work and need a specialised course. In these events, in which your motivation is partly experienced through others in the external world rather than a long-established inner drive, you may feel that you are in some sense being coerced into studying. This makes maintaining your motivation more difficult and it is a good idea to focus on what you will personally benefit from in fulfilling your study.

## Learning Aid

Avoid becoming negative and disillusioned. Focus on specific modules rather than the whole course. Try to see the positive aspects.

The general reasons for study can be seen in Box 11:1 and include both personal and professional reasons.

## Box 11:1   General Reasons for Study

**Personal**

- **Intellectual Development** – Personal growth of knowledge, skill and mind.
- **Career Advancement** – Enhances career opportunities.

*(Continued)*

- **Competition from Others** – There are now many more people who have further qualifications.

- **Employer Requirement** – Some employers may require further study and it may be necessary for specialist skills.

Professional

- **The Nature of Being a Professional** – It is part of our professional ethos to study.
- **Development of the Profession** – The profession of nursing will be better enhanced through more nurses studying.
- **Policy Changes** – Study informs the development of policies.
- **Inter-professional Necessity** – Our colleagues in the other professions are engaged in further study and we need to keep abreast of those developments.
- **Relationship between Profile and Job Description** – We need to be fit for practice in any job that we are employed to do.

# Being a Professional

It is incumbent upon the members of any profession to be highly trained, skilled and expert, and the public would not expect anything less than this. It is part of being a professional to keep abreast of the most recent advances in knowledge, certainly in their specific area of expertise, and to ensure that their practice is based on sound evidence. Whilst we would readily accept that the profession of medicine has a long history of doing this, we would have to conclude that in nursing this is a more recent emphasis. Changes in nursing occurred in the early 1980s, and although there were a number of false starts it is now clearer that being part of this professional group means that we must engage in activity that is aimed at improving the delivery of our service. We are no longer passive recipients of traditional nursing knowledge handed down from generation to generation, but proactive agents engaged in critical enquiry, research and examination of nursing action. We seek to create change through innovative practices that are rigorously tested and challenged, and we are asked to engage in intellectual reflection of our role and skills in everyday procedures. Although it is a relatively slow process, we are developing a closer relationship between academic rigour and professional nursing practice.

Another professional reason to study is the contribution that we make towards developing our profession through policy change. Through study we learn to examine issues in a more incisive manner, to analyse the implications of changing practices and to assess how alternative ways of doing things will influence patient care. Our own individual course of study may be only one small cog in a very large machine, but nonetheless it is vital that, however small, it contributes to the overall functioning of this 'machine'. This is closely related to another professional reason to study and that is a matter of inter-professional necessity. We are all aware that nursing suffers from our long-standing 'handmaiden to the medics' image, and that few would agree that nursing is on a par with medicine either as an intellectual enterprise or a scientific one. However, the modern nursing role involves intellectual debate and demands an understanding of scientific principles in order to challenge and deliberate, not only with ourselves in nursing, but also with our colleagues in the other professions. The boundaries between the many professionals in healthcare are increasingly blurred and we are duty-bound to ensure that our own functioning, as nurses, is at a high academic and practical standard.

## Learning Aid

Do not underestimate the importance of your study.

Another professional reason for studying involves the relationship between ourselves and our employers. Employers map out what they require in job specifications and seek to recruit people who appear to fit the job description. As prospective employees we attempt to become qualified and experienced enough to be successful in job applications. We need to be aware of our own individual profiles in order to know our strengths and weaknesses. This will enable us to address any gaps in our profiles and will assist us in constructing a curriculum vitae (CV) when applying for jobs. It will also be useful to map our CV against job descriptions when we are looking for employment. Box 11:2 offers you an opportunity to profile yourself against the items in it, but you can also add more for any specific areas of expertise. Studying is clearly central to many areas of this profiling exercise and if you are developing yourself and your career through the process of study then it cannot but help in the overall development of the profession.

## Box 11:2  Personal Profile

Read the items below and assess yourself in relation to the amount of skill, expertise or experience you think you have. Mark in each scale from left to right and be realistic. Example:

Once completed you will be able to see where your strengths and weaknesses are. You can now address these 'gaps' in your profile through study.

| Items | Score | |
|---|---|---|
| *Abilities* | *Minimum* | *Maximum* |

The ability to communicate in writing

The ability to communicate orally

The ability to work in a team

The ability to listen

The ability to develop relationships

The ability to solve problems

The ability to manage time effectively

The ability to self-reflect

The ability to influence others

Others (insert your own)

*Attributes*

Sharing knowledge with others

Influencing others

Networking

Negotiating

Teaching others

Flexible working

Public speaking

Attending seminars/conferences

Undertaking research

Producing publications

Having a specific area of expertise

Keeping abreast of knowledge

Academic reading

# Planning your Next Course

As is the case in many walks of life you will get out of studying what you put into it, and planning an appropriate strategy is central to making it work for you. Whatever stage you are at in your career you will probably have some idea of the general direction that you wish to pursue. However, it is unlikely that you already know exactly what each stage of your career will entail. Whatever stage you are currently at you will need to think carefully about the types of courses that you will need.

## Learning Aid

Where do I want to go? What do I want to be? When do I want to be at each stage? What courses are available?

Make sure that the course is suitable for you, and that you are suitable for the course. Choosing a course that is too advanced for you will make it difficult, unpleasant and more likely that you will fail, or fail to complete it. On the other hand, choosing a course for which you are too advanced will make this frustrating for you and you will get little benefit from it. Once you have identified your course, check where it is located and gather as much information about it as you can.

## Learning Aid

A bad course in a good institution can be as negative as a good course in a bad institution.

Ask past or present students whether they consider the course to be good or not, and ask whether they were both supported and challenged. Ask whether they benefited from attending the course and whether it lived up to expectations. Make sure that you write to the university or college and acquire a course curriculum and, once obtained, read it carefully to ensure that the content fits with your career plans. You will get the most out of your study if you find out as much as you can about your course, so attend open days and career advice centres if they have them available. Take time to walk around the campus and get a 'feel for it'. Ask yourself whether it is well signposted, whether it looks organised, what the library is like, whether it is well stocked, and so on. Are you ready for your course or do you need some preparation?

This is a very important question to ask yourself and if you answer honestly, and respond accordingly, then this will benefit you considerably. You may feel that you need a preparatory course on writing skills or to spend some time sharpening your maths skills. Some courses require you to be computer literate whilst others do not, so check out the requirements and see if you have any deficits that need addressing. You will need to ask yourself how ready you are for the course of study; Box 11:3 lists some of the main reflections.

## Box 11:3    Reflections on a Course

- Have I chosen the right course?
- Do I know the course content?
- Is it appropriate for my objectives?
- Have I considered other options?
- Did I visit the site?
- Do I have accommodation?
- Can I live there happily?
- Will I make friends?
- Do I feel ready?
- Can I afford it?
- Are there any preparatory courses to attend?
- Will I manage the course okay?
- Will it be a struggle or a challenge?
- What will be my main problems?
- How will I overcome them?
- Do I cope with anxieties well?

If you feel that you are not ready and have too many deficits then you may need to defer your course and prepare yourself more thoroughly.

## Learning Aid

Be careful that you have not underestimated yourself and that it is not merely a lack of confidence that you are feeling.

The correct balance to be achieved is a course of study that marries up to the requirements of your chosen career path, is challenging and will provide you with the correct level of knowledge and skills. If you achieve this, the major reward for you personally will be a form of enlightenment. What study does, or should do, is to produce an open mind in which you are able to appreciate many sides to an argument and appreciate many points of view. It should also enable you to produce arguments and formulate probing questions, and it should provide you with the skill to weigh the evidence appropriately and draw logical conclusions. The enlightenment it brings is to show things in a new light, to reveal hidden issues, to see tensions and conflicts, to expose dilemmas and paradoxes and to uncover the layers of human behaviour. Study is about learning what you do not know and if, at the end of a particular course of study, you *see* that you now realise that you know a lot less than you did before you started, then the study has been successful.

## Learning Aid

Read that last sentence again, carefully, and make sure that you understand it.

This brings us to our final point in this section and that is about what you get out of study in relation to the profession. If the foregoing is correct in that studying produces enlightenment, a new way of seeing things, then it will reveal the profession of nursing in a new light. If you then produce this knowledge of the profession formally, in terms of papers, policies and publications, it will contribute to the overall development of the profession. You will see nursing practice in a new way and have the skills to identify alternatives that are properly evaluated. Study will enable you to use other people's work in creative ways and to assess its impact on the profession. The relationship between study, you and the profession is a dynamic and complex one, with all aspects inextricably entwined. This dynamism involves the constant development of practice, through theory into practice and practice evaluated by theory.

## Getting out What you Put in?

General career direction.
Right course for you.
Is it a good course?
How ready are you?
Does it marry up to your career path?
Will it produce enlightenment?

## Lifelong Learning

This term is often bandied about without an understanding of its relationship both to one's personal career and to the development of the profession itself. Some view lifelong learning as a framework for undertaking course after course throughout their lives and see it merely as a personal quest for either self-fulfilment or simply to keep one's brain active. However, there is considerably more to it than that. Burgess (1997) shows that there is a complex relationship between post-graduate study, lifelong learning and a person's career. This author argues that the process of lifelong learning should be mapped out alongside a person's career and believes that graduate employment, at the required level, is closely associated with this process. Lifelong learning involves not only study on formal courses but also the informal process of learning through practice development. Some professions are better at this than others. For example, in medicine it becomes part of the ethos of the profession to be constantly engaged in learning and to improve clinical practice. As we noted above, in nursing this is a relatively new ethos for us, but one that is becoming increasingly necessary in the light of personal portfolios, PREP, fitness for practice, and so on. In fact, the English National Board (1995) clearly see lifelong learning as a complex relationship between the nurse, nursing practice, policy development, political influences, learning methods and life experiences. Box 11:4 shows the factors that the English National Board (1995) consider to be important for nurses.

## Box 11:4    Lifelong Learning (adapted from ENB, 1995)

- Practice innovation.
- Reactive to the changing demands.
- Creative learning methods.
- Accountable for their practice.
- Proactive change agents.
- Dissemination of knowledge.
- Sharing good practices.
- Responsive to changing needs.
- Challenging practices.
- Self-reliant in working practices.

## Learning throughout Life?

Map out alongside career.
Formal courses and informal learning.
Part of professional requirement.

## Career Mapping

Career mapping is concerned with strategically planning ahead of one's professional development. According to Tomey (2000: 315), 'it provides direction for formal education, experience, continuing education, professional association and networking'.

This is clearly an all-embracing definition, which means that you should consider each aspect thoroughly. This includes identifying what formal courses you will require throughout your career and what areas of work experience you wish to have. For example, following completion of your basic nursing course you may plan to study for a First Degree, then a Master's and then a PhD, and plan to specialise by working with children, which may require a further specialised course. Your plan of experience may include becoming a Health Visitor or Midwife and you may wish to gain experience working in both the community and intensive care. You will need to plan which associations you intend to join and you may wish to become a member of certain committees that focus on children's issues. You should plan which conferences you wish to attend and which individuals and organisations you should network with. Tomey (2000) suggests that careers typically move through stages, and these are: (a) exploration, (b) early career trial and establishment, (c) middle career growth and maintenance, and (d) later career plateau and decline. A career map is useful in maximising your potential and helping you to ensure that you achieve the objectives that you have set yourself.

## Thinking of a Career Map?

Formal education.
Clinical experience.
Continuing education.
Professional associations.

Your career map can be changed as you go along, and it is worthwhile revisiting it on a regular basis or in response to changing events. You need to consider what your strengths and weaknesses are and what goals you have set for yourself. Baxter (1995) outlined six groupings that he believed were helpful to people when they were choosing a career. These groupings were based on the completion of a number of short questionnaires, which were said to give an indication of the type of working style that you preferred. The groups were: (a) practical (working with things), (b) investigative (working with ideas), (c) artistic (working with ideas and people), (d) social (working with people), (e) enterprising (working with people and data) and (f) organisational/administrative (working with data and thinking). This is an interesting approach to assist you in guiding your career.

## Learning Aid

This grouping is not to be used in isolation and should only be employed alongside thorough reflection about yourself, your goals, strengths and limitations.

You should have one-year, five-year and ten-year plans within your overall career map, and an ongoing assessment of it will help you see if you are achieving your set goals. You should identify influential people who have some impact on your career and ask them to act as mentors to you.

## Changing Direction?

Develop a fluid map.
Revisit the map regularly.
One-, five- and ten-year plans.

## Learning Aid

Have business cards and swap them with colleagues. Develop your own professional library. Subscribe to at least two journals. Collect and file articles on your speciality. Chair a committee. Make presentations. Foster a support group.
Do you know the main organisations that deal with your specialist area? Who are the main people in this field?

## Career Ladders

Another helpful approach to career development is to organise a career ladder. Career ladders were developed in the 1970s, many of which were in response to the lack of career opportunities in the clinical area. Most have about four or five rungs to them to represent simple vertical advancement but they can also be constructed in many shapes and sizes to provide a more complex career structure. They can have multi-tracks and multi-levels to incorporate assessments and evaluations. For example, Tomey (2000: 308) outlines the Practice Alternatives for Career Expansion (PACE) plan, which 'is a six-level, four-track career mobility program that includes clinical, research, education and administrative tracks'. This career ladder is a sophisticated structure that incorporates behaviourally designed job descriptions as well as a performance appraisal system to evaluate progress. Illustration 11:1 shows an example of a career ladder that was designed for a ten-year career plan.

There are advantages to career ladders, and these include their potential to increase self-esteem, motivation and both personal and professional satisfaction. They can incorporate a system for rewarding certain achievements and give a clear overview of professional development. There are also a few disadvantages with career ladders, which includes their negative psychological impact when they reveal under-achievement and their use in playing one individual off against another (Tomey, 2000).

| | CLINICAL | RESEARCH | EDUCATION | ADMIN. |
|---|---|---|---|---|
| **Ten-year Evaluation Point** | Promotion | 6 Publications<br>1 Research Grant<br>2 Research Projects<br>Publication | Consider PhD | 3 Committees<br>1 Chair Exp.<br>3 Conferences |
| | Clinical Experience | Publication<br>Publication | Master's Degree | Report |
| | | Research Study | | Chair Committee |
| | Further Specialist Course | Research Grant | | |
| **Five-year Evaluation Point** | Promotion | Research Course | First Degree | Present International Conference |
| | Clinical Experience | Research Project | | Build Network |
| | Specialist Course | | | Subscribe to Two Journals |
| | Clinical Experience | Read reseach | | Present at Nursing Conference |
| | | Identify Research | | Committee Work |
| **Three-year Evaluation Point** | Complete Nursing Course | | | Subscribe to One Journal |
| | | Publication | | Build Network |
| | | | | Nursing Conference |
| | | | | Join RCN |
| **Start Point** | CLINICAL | RESEARCH | EDUCATION | ADMIN. |

**Illustration 11:1**  Career Ladders

## Learning Aid

Keep your CV 'live' by updating it regularly or as events occur.

Your CV can have multi-tracks and multi-levels.

There are advantages and disadvantages.

# Nursing Opportunities

It is difficult to imagine any profession other than medicine that has as many opportunities as does nursing. There are opportunities to nurse in-patients and out-patients, to nurse in a hospital setting or in people's homes, to nurse those at the beginning of their lives at childbirth or those approaching the end of their lives with terminal illnesses. Nurses work in industrial organisations as Occupational Health nurses as well as in the Armed Forces. They work with those vulnerable groups of people who have learning difficulties and mental health problems, as well as in schools, GP practices and prisons. Forensic nurses work with victims of sexual assault as well as with offenders who have mental health problems and have come in to contact with the law. Box 11:5 shows a list of specialist practice areas, but this list is by no means exhaustive.

## Box 11:5   Some Nursing Specialisms

Accident and Emergency

Cardiac

Intensive Care

Theatre and Anaesthetics

Older Persons

Haematology

Medical

Oncology

Paediatrics

Sexually Transmitted Diseases

Burns

*(Continued)*

*(Continued)*

Ear, Nose and Throat
Gynaecology
Obstetrics and Midwifery
Ophthalmic
Plastic Surgery
Urology
District/Community
Health Promotion
Health Visiting and Public Health
Nurse-led Community Services
Practice
School
Tropical and Refugee
Community Psychiatric
Forensic Mental Health
Learning Disabilities
Mental Health
Education
Management
Research

Not all nurses remain in clinical practice, however, and there are a number of other areas in which nurses work. Some may go into educational establishments to teach nurses in universities, colleges or their satellite schools of nursing. This is rewarding as it contributes to developing nurses and influencing the profession. Some go into research and spend their time investigating nursing practices and issues. This contributes to the development of new knowledge, and a large part of this process is applying for research funding and publishing in journals. Some nurses prefer the management career and develop their skills in this area. They aspire to management positions in which they can provide leadership qualities and influence the delivery of healthcare services. It is a demanding area to work in but highly rewarding. Finally, some nurses work for organisations such as the World Health Organisation (WHO), Nursing and Midwifery Council (NMC), Royal College of Nursing (RCN) and various aid organisations working abroad. Finally, some nurses change their careers and develop another one. This should not be viewed as negative but, on the contrary, as a positive outcome as that person is fulfilling a particular goal and will, hopefully, always carry the principles of nursing throughout their new careers.

## Looking for Nursing Opportunities?

Clinical areas are extensive.

Lecturing and teaching.

Research.

Management.

Professional associations.

# Conclusions

The main thrust of this book concerns the relationship between the skill of studying, the nurse and the profession. We have argued that studying on modern nursing courses is a skill that needs to be learnt and practised. The skill of studying can be broken down into a number of individual tasks as outlined throughout the chapters in this book, and when these are brought together they provide the framework for good scholarship. The nursing profession has changed, and is continuing to change, and it is now employing the process of learning as an active, ongoing and lifelong element of personal and professional development. We have attempted to show how study can be an enjoyable task, which is very rewarding and brings with it a sense of achievement. Throughout the book we have emphasised the point that study is as much concerned with personal development as it is with professional practice, and should be viewed as part of our professional role. It should be seen as central to our professional ethos and become a part of our everyday practice. Finally, studying should not be only about 'blood, sweat and tears' but should incorporate some element of fun. So, reward yourself for your achievements, no matter how small.

## SUMMARY POINTS OF CHAPTER 11

- Engaging in theoretical study is a crucial requisite of studying in higher education, where students can analyse the relationship between clinical practice and professional development.
- There are many benefits to undertaking studying from embarking upon the first nursing course to lifelong learning.
- The use of personal profiles allows students to examine their own skills and knowledge.
- Career mapping and career ladders are issues to be considered in lifelong learning.
- The nursing profession offers a wide range of professional opportunities, and students are encouraged to develop their strengths and ambitions from an early stage.

## Test Your Study Skills ...

1. What do you understand by lifelong learning? (see pages 198 and 206–207)

2. Why is continuing study, outside of a formal course, important to individuals and the profession? (see pages 197–198)

## Practical Session ...

1. Undertake a career-mapping exercise using a career ladder.

2. Give yourself a reward for finishing this book.

# Appendix 1: Some Definitions of Computer Language

- **ASCII (American Standard Code for Information Interchange)** – In order for information to be transferred from one computer to another standards were set. In this system the same keyboard character is represented by the same binary number on every keyboard.
- **Back-up** – This means saving your work to a hard drive and a floppy disk so that if one system fails you will still have a back-up copy.
- **Bits** – This is the smallest unit of information that a computer can hold. It contains only one of two possible binary numbers: 1 or 0 (on–off).
- **Bytes** – This refers to eight bits which are needed to represent one letter on the keyboard.
- **Cache (pronounced 'cash')** – This is a type of memory that allows information to be manipulated very fast.
- **CPU (Central Processing Unit)** – This is the brain of the computer and it both controls and executes the commands. It is often called a processor.
- **Cursor** – The point on the screen where you are working which is usually indicated by an arrow or black line. Now referred to as a 'pointer'.
- **Driver** – A software program that allows the transmission of data from your computer to another device that is connected to your computer (e.g. a printer).
- **Floppy Disk** – A small transportable disk on which you can save a relatively small amount of information. Floppy disks are used to move information between sites or to provide back-up copies of your work. They are delicate and need to be carefully handled and transported.
- **Hard Disk** – This is the main disk within your computer and can store large amounts of information. You can save your work to this disk and it is faster to work with than a floppy disk.
- **Memory** – This refers to the amount of room on a computer (or disk) that can store information. We now talk about this in terms of megabytes or gigabytes (see Box 3:1).
- **Memory Stick** – A growing number of portable devices that hold large amounts of information. They are used in cameras for digital transportation as well as PCs for transferring and holding files.

- **Modem** – This is a device that allows a computer to communicate with other computers via a telephone line. It converts the digital output of a computer to an analogue signal.
- **Mouse** – This is a device that has a small ball which when rotated moves the screen pointer around. The pointer can be located on an icon and the mouse button depressed to activate the command. This is called 'clicking the mouse'.
- **RAM (Random Access Memory)** – This is the primary working memory of the computer. When you open a program it is actually a copy that you are working on in the RAM.
- **Removable Disk** – General term for a number of disks that hold a large amount of information in various formats.
- **ROM (Read-only Memory)** – This is a permanent form of storage of information that the manufacturer of the computer puts in. You can read it but cannot write to it or save in it.

**BA (Hons)** – Bachelor of Arts university-awarded degree with honours classification. A first or basic level of degree.

**Blog** – A shortened term for web log. It is a website that functions like a personalised diary and contains images, text and commentaries on anything topical. Anyone can generate these.

**BSc (Hons)** – Bachelor of Science university-awarded degree with honours classification. A first or basic level of degree.

**CHC** – Community Health Councils are statutory bodies in England and Wales. Their function is to represent the interests of local people.

**CHI or CHIMP** – The Commission for Health Improvement is an independent statutory body that ensures standards are met.

**Clinical Governance** – This is a framework through which NHS organisations are accountable for continually improving the quality of their services.

**CPD** – Continuous Professional Development. This refers to a process by which professionals continually update and upgrade their skills, knowledge and expertise. Information for registered nurses, midwives and health visitors concerning CPD is available from the UKCC.

**CV** – A curriculum vitae is a shortened version of professional and academic qualifications, skills and expertise. Students applying for future jobs are asked to take advice from their tutors in writing their CVs. Most undergraduate courses have specific lectures that address how to write a CV.

**Degrees and Degree Classifications** – Degrees are university awards which can be classified into a number of categories. There are variations in the awarding of degrees, depending upon the institute of higher education in question. Students need to be sure what type of degree they are reading for and whether it is an honours or ordinary degree. This information can be obtained from the nursing school or department prospectus, and, in addition, students may seek further clarification from the admissions tutor or the director of studies. Most students work towards an honours degree and obtain one of the following classifications: first class (1), upper second class (2:1), lower second class (2:2) and third (3). Students must be clear as to how the marks are distributed throughout the course.

**Dip HE: Nursing Studies** – Diploma in Higher Education: Nursing Studies.

**ENB** – The English National Board, now disbanded. It had a long history of being responsible for approving the standards of higher education institutions and their courses of study.

**Evidence-based Practice, Evidence-based Medicine and Evidence-based Healthcare** – There is no specific definition for any of these terms, but they bring together a number of fundamental ideas and concepts. This includes the application of a scientific approach to decision-making, policies and the delivery of care to patients and clients.

**Formative Evaluation** – An evaluation which takes place throughout the course or learning experience.

**HAZ** – Health Action Zone is a district with significant inequalities in health.

**MA** – Master of Arts. A higher degree awarded by a university.

**MSc** – Master of Science. A higher degree awarded by a university.

**NHSnet** – The health services' information superhighway. This service carries clinical information across the country.

**NICE** – The National Institute for Clinical Excellence has been set up to promote clinical standards and cost-effectiveness in the NHS. It has an advisory role for practice and appraises original technologies and treatments. NICE works to promote geographical equity and evidence-based practice.

**NMC** – The Nursing and Midwifery Council. This is the regulatory body of nurses and midwives, superseding the UKCC. The NMC is responsible for the quality and assurance of education programmes leading to registration and recordable qualifications. The NMC focuses on public protection through the regulation of its members.

The address of the NMC is 23 Portland Place, London, W1B 1PZ. Email address: www.nmc–uk.org

**NSFs** – National Service Frameworks establish national standards for services in major areas or disease groups.

**NT** – *Nursing Times* is the most widely read nursing journal in the United Kingdom today.

**OSCEs** – Objective Structural Clinical Exams

**PhD** – Doctor of Philosophy. A higher degree of study, usually research-based, in which new and original knowledge must be produced.

**Podcast** – This is a digital media file, accessed through the Internet, to be played back on portable media players, etc.

**PPP** – Personal Professional Profiles must be used by nurses to document their relevant learning activity; they can be designed and put together by nurses themselves, or nurses can obtain specially designed PPPs, often from their employers.

**PREP** – Post-registration Education and Practice is a set of NMC standards that nurses must meet to show that they have maintained and developed their professional knowledge and competence. To stay on the register (able to practise nursing) nurses need, first to complete a notification of practice form when they re-register every three years and/or when they change their area of professional practice to one where they will use a different register qualification. Second, nurses must complete 35 hours of learning activity every three years. Third, nurses must maintain a personal professional profile containing details of continuing professional development, and fourth, nurses must comply with any request from the NMC to audit the way they have met these requirements.

**Summative Evaluation** – An evaluation which takes place at the end of the course or learning experience.

**Tutors: Personal and Academic** – Each student is allocated at least one tutor at the beginning of their course of study. Some institutions, usually the older universities, will allocate students two tutors. This will include an academic tutor from within the department and a personal tutor from outside the department. The rationale for this is for students' personal and academic issues to be kept separate and by having a personal tutor from another school or department they may feel more at ease in discussing any personal problems that they may have. Other institutions allocate students just one tutor who acts as both academic and personal tutor. The rationale for this is to enable tutors to have a greater overview of their students' progress, which may be affected by personal issues. It also allows students and tutors to get to know each other.

**UKCC** – The United Kingdom Central Council was the regulatory body for nurses, midwives and health visitors. The UKCC has been superseded by the NMC (The Nursing and Midwifery Council). See NMC above.

# Further Reading

## General

Baddeley, A. (2004) *Your Memory: A User's Guide.* London: Prion.

Bourner, T. and Race, P. (1990) *How to Win as a Part-time Student.* London: Kogan Page.

Crème, P. and Lea, M.R. (1997) *Writing at University: A Guide for Students.* Milton Keynes: Open University Press.

Fink, A. (2004) *Conducting Research Literature Reviews from the Internet to Paper.* London: Sage

Hart, C. (1998) *Doing a Literature Review: Releasing the Social Science Research Imagination.* London: Sage.

Hart, C. (2001) *Doing a Literature Search: A Comprehensive Guide for the Social Sciences.* London: Sage.

Northedge, A., Thomas, J., Lane, A. and Peasgood, A. (1997) *The Sciences Good Study Guide.* Milton Keynes: Open University Press.

Redman, P. (2005) *Good Essay Writing.* London: Sage.

Turner, J. (2002) *How to Study: A Short Introduction.* London: Sage.

## Healthcare

Burns, S. and Bulman, C. (2000) *Reflective Practice in Nursing: The Growth of the Professional Practitioner* (2nd edn). Oxford: Blackwell Science.

Castledine, G. (1998) *Writing, Documentation and Communication for Nurses.* Dinton, Wiltshire: Mark Allen.

Maslin-Prothero, S. (2001) *Baillière's Study Skills for Nurses* (2nd edn). Edinburgh/London: Baillière Tindall/Royal College of Nursing.

Porter, M.E. and Teisberg, E.O. (2006) *Redefining Health Care: Creating Value-based Competition on Results.* Boston: Harvard Business School.

Taylor, B.J. (2000) *Reflective Practice: A Guide for Nurses and Midwives.* Buckingham: Open University Press.

Winters, J. (1995) *Practical Study Skills for Nurses.* London: Scutari Press.

Wurman, R.S. (2004) *Understanding Healthcare.* London: Johnson & Johnson

## Critique

Brink-Budgen, R. van den (1999) *Critical Thinking for Students* (2nd edn). Oxford: How To Books.

Crombie, I.K. (1996) *Critical Appraisal.* London: BMJ Publishing Group.

Moore, B.N. and Parker, R. (2005) *Critical Thinking 8th Edition*. Maidenhead: McGraw Hill.

## Dyslexic Students

Miles, T.R. and Gilroy, D.E. (1995) *Dyslexia at College* (2nd edn). London: Routledge.

Shaywitz, S. (2005) *Overcoming Dyslexia: A New and Complete Science-based Program for Reading Problems at Any Level*. London: Vintage.

## Information Technology

Bower, A.G. (2005) *The Diffusion and Value of Healthcare Information Technology*. Cambridge: Rand Health Corporation.

Honeycutt, J. (1996) *Using the Internet* (2nd edn). Indianapolis: Que Corporation.

Nicoll, L.H. (2001) *Nurses' Guide to the Internet* (3rd edn). Philadelphia: Lippincott.

Thede, L.Q. (1999) *Computers in Nursing: Bridges to the Future*. Philadelphia: Lippincott.

## Reflection

Benner, P. (1984) *From Novice to Expert: Excellence and Power in Clinical Nursing Practice*. London: Addison-Wesley.

Bolton, G.E.J. (2005) *Reflective Practice: Writing and Professional Development*. London: Sage.

Boud, D., Keogh, R. and Walker, D. (1985) *Reflection: Turning Experience into Learning*. London: Kogan Page.

Brown, J. (2006) *A Leader's Guide to Reflective Practice*. Oxford: Trafford Publishing.

Moon, J. (1999) *Reflection in Learning and Professional Development*. London: Kogan Page.

Rolfe, G. (1997) Beyond expertise: theory, practice and the reflective practitioner. *Journal of Clinical Nursing*, 6: 93–7.

Schon, D. (1983) *The Reflective Practitioner: How Professionals Think in Action*. New York: Basic Books.

Schon, D. (1987) *Educating the Reflective Practitioner: Towards a New Design for Teaching and Learning in the Professions*. San Francisco: Jossey-Bass.

# References

Andrews, M.M. (1999) How to search for information on transcultural nursing and health subjects: Internet and CD-ROM sources. *Journal of Transcultural Nursing*, 10(1): 69–74.

Baxter, R. (1995) *Studying Successfully.* Richmond: Aldbrough St John Publications.

Borton, T. (1970) *Reach, Teach and Touch.* London: McGraw Hill.

Boud, D., Keogh, R. and Walker, D. (1985) *Reflection: Turning Experience into Learning.* London: Kogan Page.

Boyd, E. and Fales, A. (1983) Reflective learning: key to learning from experience. *Journal of Humanistic Psychology*, 23(2): 99–117.

Breslow, R.A., Ross, S.A. and Weed, D.L. (1998) Public health briefs: quality of reviews in epidemiology. *American Journal of Public Health*, 88(3): 474–7.

Burden, B. (2001) Writing a review of the literature: a practical guide. *British Journal of Midwifery*, 9(8): 498–501.

Burgess, R. (1997) *Beyond the First Degree: Graduate Education, Lifelong Learning and Careers.* Buckingham: Open University Press.

Burns, S. and Bulman, C. (2000) *Reflective Practice in Nursing: The Growth of the Professional Practitioner* (2nd edn). Oxford: Blackwell Science.

Campbell, P. (1998) Listening to clients. In P.J. Barker and B. Davidson (eds), *Ethical Strife.* London: Arnold.

Daloz, L.A. (1986) *Effective Teaching and Mentoring.* London: Jossey-Bass.

Data Protection Act (1998) London: The Stationery Office.

Dewey, J. (1933) *How We Think: A Restatement of the Relation of Reflective Thinking to the Educative Process.* Boston, MA: D.C. Heath.

Disability Discrimination Act (1995) London: The Stationery Office.

Education Act (1994) London: The Stationery Office.

English National Board (1990) *Regulations & Guidelines for the Approval of Institutions and Courses.* London: ENB.

English National Board (1995) *Creating Lifelong Learners: Partnerships for Care: Guidelines for the Implementation of the UKCC's Standards for Education and Practice following Registration.* London: ENB.

Further and Higher Education Act (1992) London: The Stationery Office.

Greaves, F. (1984) *Nurse Education and the Curriculum.* London: Croom Helm.

Green, B.N., Johnson, C.D. and Adams, A. (2000) Writing narrative literature reviews for peer reviewed journals: secrets of the trade. *Journal of Sports Chiropractic and Rehabilitation*, 15(1): 5–19.

Hobbes, T. ([1651] 1976) *Leviathan.* Harmondsworth: Penguin.

Johns, C. (2000) *Becoming a Reflective Practitioner: A Reflective & Holistic Approach to Clinical Nursing, Practice Development & Clinical Supervision.* Oxford: Blackwell.

Kember, D. (2001) *Reflective Teaching and Learning in the Health Professions.* Oxford: Blackwell Science.

Kratz, C.R. (1979) *The Nursing Process.* London: Ballière Tindall.

Lorig, K. (2000) *Patient Education: A Practical Approach*. London: Sage.

Lutters, M. and Vogt, N. (2000) What is the basis for treating infections your way? *Journal of the American Geriatrics Society*, 48(11): 1454–61.

Nachmias, C. and Nachmias, D. (1981) *Research Methods in the Social Sciences*. London: Edward Arnold.

NHS CRD (National Health Service Centre for Reviews and Dissemination) (2001) *Undertaking Systematic Reviews of Research on Effectiveness*. York: University of York Press.

Parnes, S.J., Noller, R.B. and Biondi, A.M. (1977) *Guide to Creative Action: Revised Edition of Creative Behavior Guidebook*. New York: Scribner.

Roper, N., Logan, W.W. and Tierney, A.J. (1996) *The Elements of Nursing: A Model for Nursing Based on a Model of Living* (4th edn). London: Churchill Livingstone.

Schon, D. (1983) *The Reflective Practitioner: How Professionals Think in Action*. New York: Basic Books.

Schon, D. (1987) *Educating the Reflective Practitioner: Towards a New Design for Teaching and Learning in the Professions*. San Francisco: Jossey-Bass.

Snider, L. (2000) Evidence-based practice: reviewing qualitative research. *Occupational Therapy Now*, 2(5): 5–6.

Special Educational Needs and Disability Act (2001) London: The Stationery Office.

Taylor, B.J. (2000) *Reflective Practice: A Guide for Nurses and Midwives*. Buckingham: Open University Press.

Thede, L.Q. (1999) *Computers in Nursing: Bridges to the Future*. Philadelphia: Lippincott.

Tomey, A.M. (2000) *Guide to Nursing Management and Leadership* (6th edn). St Louis: Mosby.

Wilkie, A. (2000) The nature of problem-based learning in nursing. In S. Glen and K. Wilkie (eds), *Problem-based Learning in Nursing*. London: Macmillan.

# Index